Mosby's Workbook for

The Homemaker/Home Health Aide

by Julie Wernig
Sheila A. Sorrentino

Mary Heath, R.N., B.S.N.
Health Education Instructor,
St. James Hospital;
former Coordinator and Instructor,
Practical Nursing Program,
Kankakee Community College;
Pontiac, Illinois

The C.V. Mosby Company
* St. Louis * Toronto * Baltimore * 1989

Editor-in-chief: David T. Culverwell
Editorial Project Manager: Lisa G. Cunninghis
Composition/Project Management: The Production House

Copyright © 1989 by The C.V. Mosby Company

Printed in the United States of America

All rights reserved. Except in classes in which *The Homemaker/Home Health Aide* by Julie Wernig and Sheila Sorrentino is used, no part of this publication may be reproduced, stored in a retrieval system, or transmitted, in any form or by any means, electronic, mechanical, photocopying, recording, or otherwise, without prior written permission from the publisher.

The C.V. Mosby Company
11830 Westline Industrial Drive
St. Loius, Missouri 63146

ISBN 0-8016-5529-3

PH/VH/VH 9 8 7 6 5 4 3 2

PREFACE

Mosby's Workbook for The Homemaker/ Home Health Aide is intended to be used as a learning tool for the student who is using *Mosby's Textbook for The Homemaker/ Home Health Aide*. The workbook has been designed with a variety of exercises and activities for the student to complete after studying the corresponding chapter in the text.

Key terms from each chapter are highlighted in "Terms to Know." In several chapters, a section entitled "Checking Up on Procedures" asks the student to number essential steps from a specific procedure in order. This encourages the student to think about the actions performed and logically number them. Due to the length of certain procedures, not all steps in a procedure are included. Other sections ask the student to decide if an action is safe or unsafe or to tell how frequently housekeeping tasks need to be performed in the client's home. Crossword and Hidden Word puzzles are used to enhance spelling as well as meaning. Diagrams, sketches, and pictures of equipment are included for labeling. "Fill-in" and "List" sections emphasize information that the student needs to be able to recall from memory.

The answers to the chapter questions are found in the back of the book so that the student can work independently and can study correct information, not errors. A final Examination is included, which covers the entire text. This may serve as a means of preparing for an end-of-course evaluation or as a review.

CONTENTS

1	Introduction to Home Care 1		10	Body Mechanics 39
2	The Home Health Aide 4		11	Activity 44
3	Communicating Effectively 7		12	Bedmaking 48
4	Communicating in the Home Health Agency 10		13	Vital Signs 52
			14	Personal Care 59
5	Understanding the Needs of Clients 15		15	Elimination 64
6	Understanding How the Body Functions 18		16	Collecting Specimens 69
			17	Food and Fluids 74
7	Controlling Infection in the Home 29		18	Special Procedures 78
8	Safety 33		19	The Postoperative Client 82
9	Home Maintenance 36		20	The Mother and Her Newborn . . . 86

21	Common Health Problems 90	Final Examination 103
22	Basic Emergency Care 95	Answers to Chapter Questions 118
23	The Dying Client. 100	

CHAPTER 1

Introduction to Home Care

TERMS TO KNOW Using the list below, write the term on the line with the correct definition.

diagnostic related group
health maintenance organization
home health aide
homebound
homemaker

hospice
Medicaid
Medicare
plan of treatment
policy and procedure manual

_____ 1. A federally funded health insurance program for the elderly

_____ 2. A written plan signed by the doctor that describes the client's plan for home care

_____ 3. Confined to the home

_____ 4. A program for persons dying of terminal illnesses

_____ 5. A method of paying hospitals for Medicare and Medicaid clients

_____ 6. A health insurance plan sponsored by federal and state governments for the poor, elderly, blind, and disabled and for families with dependent children

_____ 7. A prepaid group insurance plan that provides a wide range of services to meet a client's total health care needs

_____ 8. A health care worker who helps the client and family maintain the home

_____ 9. A health care worker who provides personal care, comfort, and housekeeping services

_____ 10. A manual that describes how the agency operates and how procedures are to be done

TRUE AND FALSE

Mark the statement "T" for true or "F" for false. Change the false statements to make them true.

_____ 1. Home care is usually more expensive than hospital care.
_____ 2. People of all ages and income levels can benefit from home care.
_____ 3. Home health services help the client or family maintain the home.
_____ 4. Under Medicaid, monthly premiums are paid by those insured.
_____ 5. The responsibilities of each position in an agency are explained in the job description.
_____ 6. Personnel policies describe specific standards for client care.
_____ 7. Home care promotes self-care, independence, and dignity.
_____ 8. Diagnostic related groups (DRGs) were legislated by Congress to help reduce Medicare and Medicaid costs.
_____ 9. A client's questions about payment for home care services should be answered by the doctor.
_____ 10. Most home care clients are elderly.

MULTIPLE CHOICE

Select the correct word or group of words in parentheses to complete each statement.

1. A client who suffers from an illness from which there is no reasonable expectation for recovery is said to have a (*chronic, terminal*) illness.
2. An agency's (*organizational chart, policy and procedure manual*) shows lines of authority and responsibility.
3. The home health aide works under the supervision of the (*licensed practical nurse, registered nurse*).
4. The plan of treatment for client care is developed and changed as needed by the (*supervisor, director, doctor*).
5. Exercises and treatments to restore function to a body part are provided by the (*physical therapist, occupational therapist, respiratory therapist*).
6. Clients or families with social or psychological problems may be counseled by the (*speech pathologist, social worker, supervisor*).
7. A prepaid group insurance plan that provides a wide range of services to meet a client's total health care needs is called a/an (*HHA, HMO, PPO*).

INTRODUCTION TO HOME CARE

CROSSWORD PUZZLE

Complete the crossword puzzle by identifying the members of the home care team from the clues below.

Across:
2. Counsels and instructs in nutrition, food prepparation, and special diets
4. An RN who assigns and supervises the activities of other RNs, LPNs, home health aides, and homemakers
7. Gives breathing treatments, evaluates breathing, and checks respiratory equipment in the home
8. Gives personal care, performs simple nursing procedures, gives emotional comfort, provides housekeeping services, reports and records changes in the client's condition
9. Does basic housekeeping tasks; may provide child care
10. Helps find community services or organizations which meet the needs of the client and the family

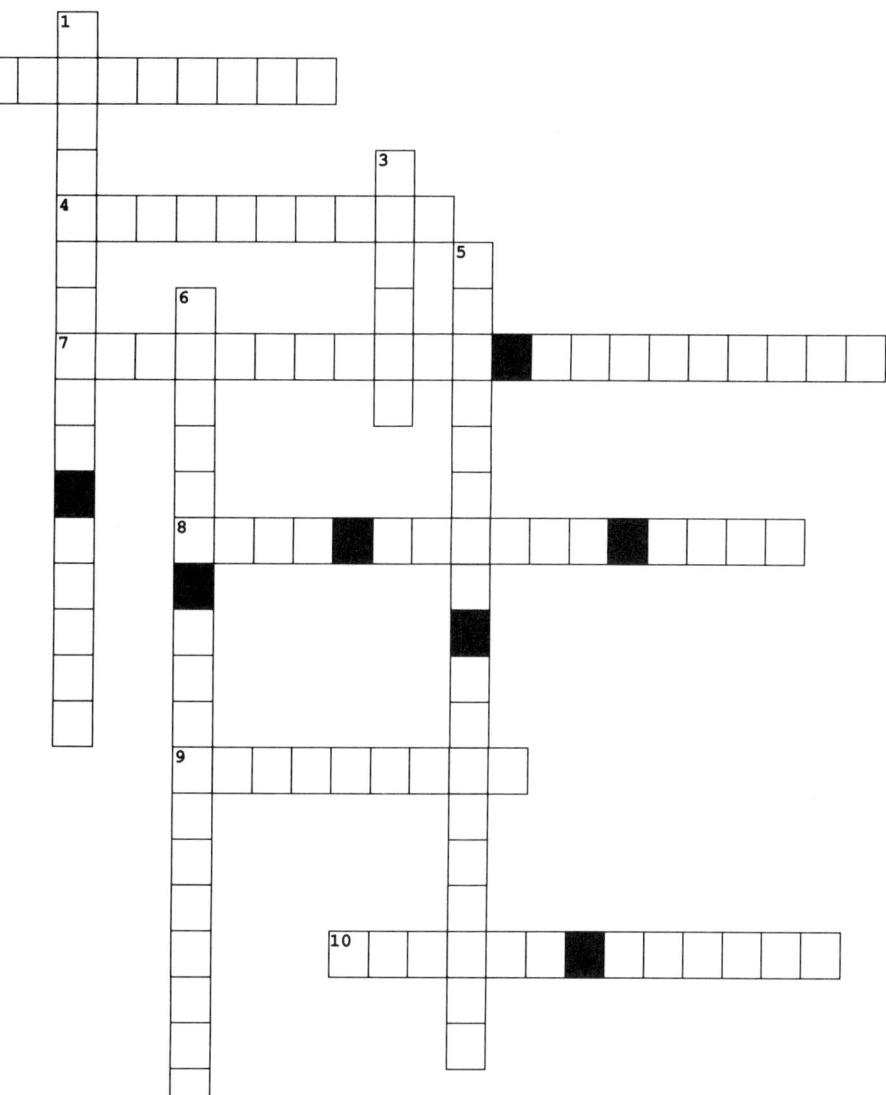

Down:
1. Assesses, plans, implements, and evaluates care while carrying out doctor's orders
3. Diagnoses, prescribes, and treats clients; develops and changes the treatment plan as needed
5. Provides treatments and exercises that help restore function or prevent disability
6. Treats clients with speech, language, or swallowing disorders

CHAPTER 2

The Home Health Aide

TERMS TO KNOW

Match the terms listed in Column A with the correct definition from Column B.

Column A

____ 1. Assault
____ 2. Battery
____ 3. Confidentiality
____ 4. Ethics
____ 5. False imprisonment
____ 6. Incident
____ 7. Negligence
____ 8. Will

Column B

a. An accident or unusual occurrence
b. Standards for behavior
c. Threatening or attempting to touch a person's body without consent
d. Keeping client information private
e. A legal document that states what should be done with money and property after death
f. Touching a person without consent
g. Restricting a person's movements without consent
h. The unintentional harming of another person or their property

UNDERSTANDING ROLES AND RESPONSIBILITIES

Mark each statement with "YES" if it describes a task that a home health aide is expected to perform. Mark the statement "NO" if it describes a task that a home health aide should not perform.

____ 1. Assist with bathing and mouth care
____ 2. Prepare meals
____ 3. Give oral medications
____ 4. Measure vital signs
____ 5. Collect specimens
____ 6. Supervise the work of another home health aide
____ 7. Record activities and observations of the client

THE HOME HEALTH AIDE

_____ 8. Record a telephone order from the doctor
_____ 9. Assist with transfers
_____ 10. Inform the client's family of the treatment plan
_____ 11. Perform sterile dressing changes
_____ 12. Ignore any request to perform a task for which you have not been prepared

TRUE AND FALSE

Mark the statement "T" for true or "F" for false. Change the false statements to make them true.

_____ 1. Right to privacy means the right to have confidential information revealed.
_____ 2. Money and family problems of the client are examples of confidential information.
_____ 3. Gossiping about clients or their families is considered unethical behavior.
_____ 4. You should be given a written copy of your job description shortly after you start to work.
_____ 5. Unintentionally harming a client or a client's property is called battery.
_____ 6. You can be sued in a court of law for negligence.
_____ 7. An incident is an accident or unusual occurrence that involves the client only.
_____ 8. When an incident occurs, you should report it at the end of your shift.
_____ 9. When completing an incident report, you should not give opinions; just state the facts.
_____ 10. You may help a client with the wording of their will.

MULTIPLE CHOICE

Select the correct word or group of words in parentheses to complete each statement.

1. Being aware of the needs, feelings, likes, and dislikes of others is called (_flexibility, empathy, sensitivity_).
2. Performing duties to the best of one's ability is known as (_self-awareness, consideration, conscientiousness_).
3. Home health aides (_may, may not_) wear colored nail polish to work.
4. You are unsure about a procedure you are to perform. You should ask for help from (_your supervisor, the doctor, the client's family_).
5. Most agencies allow employees to wear (_regular clothing, wedding rings, jewelry of any type_).

6. Forcing an unwilling client to take a bath would be considered (*assault, battery, negligence*).
7. To restrain a client in bed without a doctor's order is called (*negligence, battery, false imprisonment*).
8. (*All, many*) states have laws which require training for home health aides.
9. An incident occurs in the home. You need to complete an incident report. (*Do, do not*) write in the client's chart that an incident report has been filed.
10. Individuals who are named in a will (*can, cannot*) witness its signing.

LIST

1. List four questions you can ask yourself to help decide if an action is ethical or unethical.

    a. _____
    b. _____
    c. _____
    d. _____

2. Give two examples of unethical behavior:

    a. _____
    b. _____

3. Give two examples of negligent acts:

    a. _____
    b. _____

4. Give two examples of incidents in the home that need to be reported:

    a. _____
    b. _____

CHAPTER 3
Communicating Effectively

TERMS TO KNOW

Supply the correct term from the list to complete the sentences below.

body language   nonverbal communication   cliché
communication   verbal communication   tact
feedback

1. The giving and receiving of information by two or more people is called _____.
2. Through _____ _____, messages are sent by using facial expressions, gestures, and posture.
3. A _____ is a pat answer or common expression.
4. The sending of messages without the use of words is known as _____ _____.
5. _____ _____ occurs when words and language are used to exchange information.
6. Thinking before you act or speak and trying to say and do the right thing at the right time is known as _____.
7. A way to check communication is by receiving _____.

TRUE AND FALSE

Mark the statement "T" for true or "F" for false. Change the false statements to make them true.

_____ 1. Besides body language, verbal communication involves such things as touch, tone of voice, and smells.

_____ 2. Verbal and nonverbal communication can occur at the same time.

_____ 3. Verbal messages more accurately indicate how a person feels.

_____ 4. Being judgmental or giving opinions to clients may cause a barrier to communication with them.

_____ 5. Communicating with clients and their families is the same as talking to friends.

_____ 6. Touch can be a very simple way of communicating to someone that you care about them.

_____ 7. If a client continually refuses to see even close relatives, you must tell the relatives not to visit.

_____ 8. Always knock and announce your presence before entering a client's room.

_____ 9. Tension and conflict within a family usually improves while the client is ill.

_____ 10. You are uncomfortable with the way a family member treats the client. Discussing your feelings and concerns with that family member may be helpful.

COMMUNICATING EFFECTIVELY

The following are examples of situations you might encounter while caring for clients. Place a check on the line if the example shows good communication. Think about each situation and decide how you would handle it. Can you find any examples of communication barriers?

_____ 1. You are not certain what Mr. S. has just told you. You reply, "I'm not sure I heard what you said. Could you repeat that?"

_____ 2. Mrs. J. says she does not feel like getting dressed today. You respect her wishes and leave her alone.

_____ 3. Mrs. R. says she has nothing to live for and would rather be dead. You tell her she looks much better today, and you ask her if she has read the paper.

_____ 4. Mr. B. has been having trouble with his daughter. You tell him he should not let her come to visit so frequently.

_____ 5. You are not able to answer Mr. T.'s question about his new medicine. You tell him you will ask your supervisor to talk with him about it tomorrow.

_____ 6. Your new client resents having you in his home. You perform his care and leave as quickly as possible.

_____ 7. You are caring for Mrs. M. who is dying. One day she seems very frightened and is crying. You hold her hand and sit with her until her son arrives.

_____ 8. While visiting with friends, Mr. W. becomes very tired. You ask his friends if they could visit at another time and suggest that Mr. W. needs to rest.

_____ 9. Mrs. V.'s new hairstyle is very unattractive, but you tell her she looks wonderful.

_____ 10. Mrs. P.'s daughter stops by every morning and prevents you from caring for her mother until she leaves. You tell your supervisor about the interruptions.

_____ 11. Your client makes an unkind remark about an organization to which you belong. You do not respond to the remark, nor do you let the client know about your membership.

_____ 12. Mr. A. is very hard of hearing. When you talk to him, you must shout in his good ear.

CHAPTER 4

Communicating in the Home Health Agency

TERMS TO KNOW Match the terms listed in Column A with the correct definition from Column B.

Column A

_____ 1. Care plan
_____ 2. Symptom
_____ 3. Abbreviation
_____ 4. Prefix
_____ 5. Suffix
_____ 6. Sign
_____ 7. Client record
_____ 8. Root

Column B

a. The main part of a word
b. The written account of a client's care
c. An observed change in a client's condition
d. A written plan that lists the client's problems, goals, and activities
e. A shortened word
f. A word element placed at the end of a word
g. Something the client feels that you cannot see, hear, feel, or smell
h. A word element placed at the beginning of a word

FORMING MEDICAL TERMS Find the list of common roots in your text (pp. 29–30). Use the correct prefix from the list (pp. 27–28) to form the medical terms that mean the following:

1. difficult breathing   _____
2. within the vein   _____
3. excessive thyroid   _____
4. rapid heart   _____

10

COMMUNICATING IN THE HOME HEALTH AGENCY 11

5. much urine _____
6. across the abdomen _____
7. inside the heart _____

Now use the list of suffixes (p. 30) with the correct root to form the medical terms that mean the following:

8. liver enlargement _____
9. throat inflammation _____
10. removal of the breast _____
11. nerve tumor _____
12. head pain _____
13. excessive blood flow _____
14. creation of an opening in the stomach _____
15. surgical reshaping of the nose _____
16. examination of the bronchus using a scope _____

CLIENT RECORDS

It is important to know where to find information in the client's record. The various chart forms are listed below. Place the letter of each form on the lines to indicate where you can find the information needed. You will use some forms more than once.

a. graphic sheet
b. nursing notes
c. care plan
d. ADL sheet
e. work plan
f. physician order sheet
g. initial assessment
h. client information

_____ 1. Medication orders
_____ 2. Client's age and birthdate
_____ 3. TPR
_____ 4. Problems and goals for the client's condition
_____ 5. Allergies of the client
_____ 6. Who will perform certain tasks for the client
_____ 7. A record of observations and treatments as well as the client's response to care
_____ 8. Names, addresses, and phone numbers of persons to contact in an emergency
_____ 9. The amount of assistance the client needs to complete daily functions such as bathing and toileting

_____ 10. BP
_____ 11. Week-long assignment of household duties
_____ 12. Habits and preferences of a new client

MULTIPLE CHOICE Select the correct word or group of words in parentheses to complete each statement.

1. A (*sign, symptom*) is a change in the client's condition that you can see, hear, feel, or smell.
2. (*Objective, subjective*) recording is using the client's own words to describe what he or she feels.
3. All entries in the client's record should be made with (*pencil, red ink, black ink*).
4. Chart at least every (*two, four, eight*) hours.
5. The best time to make observations about a client is when (*the client is sleeping, giving personal care, the client has visitors*).
6. When recording the client's own words, be sure to (*underline, use quotation marks, use red ink*).
7. If a task is not charted, it is assumed that it (*was, was not*) completed.
8. If you make an error in charting, (*draw a line through the wrong entry and write "error," white out the error, start a new entry*).
9. You (*may, may not*) chart activities performed by another person.
10. When charting, (*avoid, use*) words such as "normal," "good," or "adequate."

MATCHING *Part 1.* Match the common root in Column A with the correct meaning in Column B.

Column A
_____ 1. Crani(o)
_____ 2. Gastr(o)
_____ 3. Hemat(o)
_____ 4. Nephr(o)
_____ 5. Ocul(o)
_____ 6. Psych(o)
_____ 7. Stomat(o)
_____ 8. Thromb(o)
_____ 9. Urin(o)
_____ 10. Uter(o)

Column B
a. Uterus
b. Clot, thrombus
c. Kidney
d. Mind
e. Skull
f. Blood
g. Stomach
h. Urine
i. Mouth
j. Eye

Part 2. Match the abbreviation in Column A with the correct meaning in Column B.

	Column A		Column B
_____	11. ad lib	a.	Four times a day
_____	12. bid	b.	Drops
_____	13. BRP	c.	Nothing by mouth
_____	14. gtt	d.	As desired
_____	15. NKA	e.	Three times a day
_____	16. NPO	f.	Both eyes
_____	17. OD	g.	Bathroom privileges
_____	18. OS	h.	As needed
_____	19. OU	i.	Twice a day
_____	20. prn	j.	Left eye
_____	21. qid	k.	No known allergies
_____	22. tid	l.	Right eye

CROSSWORD PUZZLE

Complete the crossword puzzle by identifying the meanings for the abbreviations given in the clues below.

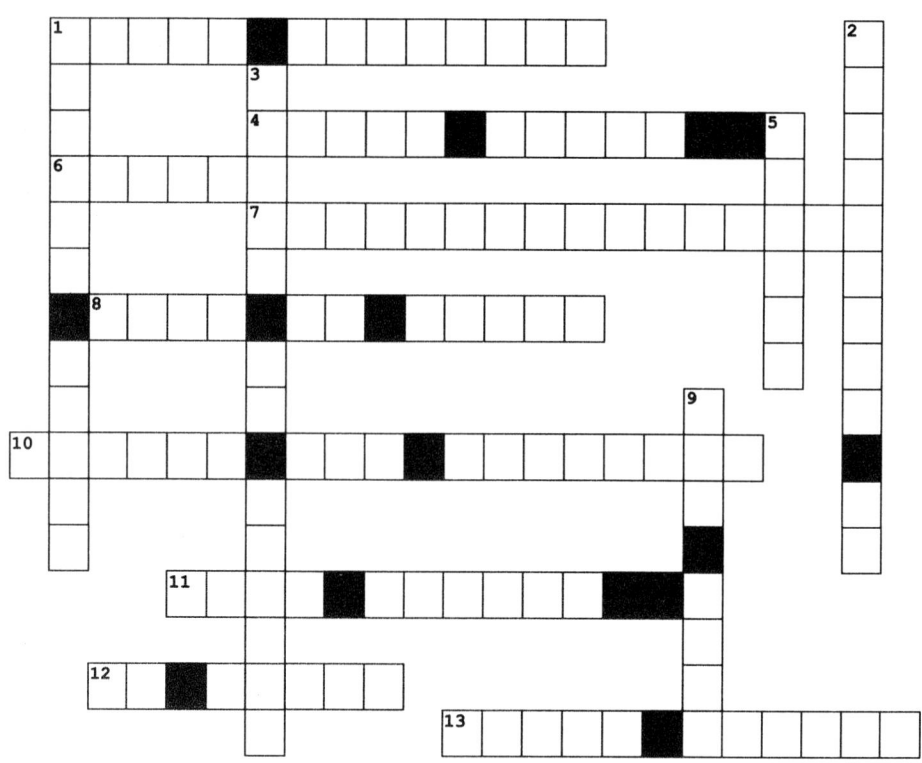

Across:

1. BM
4. p.c.
6. O_2
7. G.I.
8. HS
10. N/V
11. VS
12. po
13. FF

Down:

1. a.c.
2. c/o
3. ROM
5. CA
9. ss

CHAPTER 5
Understanding the Needs of Clients

TERMS TO KNOW Using the list below, write the term on the line with the correct definition.

aging
bias
culture
disability
esteem

extended family
menarche
menopause
need

nuclear family
puberty
self-esteem
sexuality

_____ 1. Permanent loss of a physical or mental function

_____ 2. When menstruation stops

_____ 3. Physical, psychological, social, cultural, and spiritual factors which affect a person's feelings and attitudes about his or her sex

_____ 4. That which is required or desirable for life and mental well-being

_____ 5. When a person thinks that he or she is a worthwhile and valuable person

_____ 6. The nuclear family plus grandparents, aunts, uncles, and cousins

_____ 7. When reproductive organs begin to function and secondary sex characteristics appear

_____ 8. The start of menstruation

_____ 9. An unfavorable opinion, judgment, or attitude

_____ 10. Worth and value

_____ 11. Values, beliefs, and customs that are passed down from one generation to the next

_____ 12. Mother, father, and children who live together

_____ 13. The process of growing older

TRUE AND FALSE

Mark the statement "T" for true or "F" for false. Change the false statements to make them true.

_____ 1. Lower level needs must be met before higher level needs.
_____ 2. Examples of physical needs include the need for affection, and for being cared about and wanted by others.
_____ 3. Learning as much as possible about a client's culture can help you avoid becoming biased.
_____ 4. Young adulthood is the time between 12 and 18 years of age.
_____ 5. Sex takes on more meaning as young adults mature.
_____ 6. Sometimes sexually aggressive behaviors are due to confusion or disorientation.
_____ 7. An increase in appetite is known as anorexia.
_____ 8. Signs and symptoms of disease occur very slowly in children.
_____ 9. The elderly are the main users of home care services.
_____ 10. Blindness, deafness, mental retardation, and speech disorders are examples of disabilities.

GROWTH AND DEVELOPMENT

Using the code below, mark each statement to identify the stage of development described.

a. infancy
b. toddler
c. preschool
d. school age
e. adolescence
f. young adulthood
g. adulthood
h. late adulthood

_____ 1. Menopause occurs in women
_____ 2. Asks questions about everything; needs simple answers
_____ 3. Learns by sucking, touching, and looking at things
_____ 4. Begins to develop morals, values, and a conscience
_____ 5. Full physical growth and development reached
_____ 6. Illness and disease are common
_____ 7. Starts toilet training
_____ 8. Puberty occurs
_____ 9. Temper tantrums occur
_____ 10. Develops an identity
_____ 11. Begins to trust others
_____ 12. Uses imagination in play; may have imaginary playmate

___ 13. Emotional reactions are hard to control
___ 14. Few illnesses or health problems
___ 15. Becomes involved in group activities; plays team sports

FILL IN Complete this chart by supplying the missing information.

Stage	Age	Examples of Toy/Activity For Age
	0–1	
Toddler		
		Puzzles, trucks, dolls, tricycles
	6–12	
Adolescence		

MULTIPLE CHOICE Select the correct word or group of words in parentheses to complete each statement.

1. During (*infancy, toddlerhood*) rapid physical, psychological, and social growth occurs.
2. Learning to judge right from wrong is a task of children of the (*preschool, school, adolescent*) age group.
3. Friends or peers are very important in the life of the (*preschool, school*) age child.
4. The elderly person needs (*more, less*) sleep than during the younger years.
5. Fears about monsters, ghosts, and boogeymen are common in children of (*infancy, toddler, preschool*) age.
6. After (*menarche, menopause*) a women can no longer have children.
7. Sexuality is present from (*birth, puberty, adolescence*) on.

CHAPTER 6

Understanding How the Body Functions

TERMS TO KNOW Match the term listed in Column A with the correct definition found in Column B.

Part 1. *Column A* *Column B*
_____ 1. Cell a. The cell's control center
_____ 2. Protoplasm b. Groups of cells
_____ 3. Nucleus c. Groups of tissues
_____ 4. Tissues d. Basic unit of the body
_____ 5. Organs e. Organs that work together
_____ 6. System f. Living matter within cells

Part 2. *Column A* *Column B*
_____ 1. Neuron a. Controls heart rate, breathing, vomiting
_____ 2. Cerebrum b. Three-layer covering of brain and spinal cord
_____ 3. Cerebellum c. The nerve cell
_____ 4. Brainstem d. Largest part of the brain
_____ 5. Spinal cord e. Controls movement and balance
_____ 6. Meninges f. Contains paths to send messages to and from brain

Part 3. *Column A* *Column B*
_____ 1. Plasma a. Carry blood away from heart
_____ 2. Systole b. Carry blood to heart
_____ 3. Diastole c. Liquid part of blood

UNDERSTANDING HOW THE BODY FUNCTIONS

    ____ 4. Arteries   d. Very tiny connecting vessels
    ____ 5. Capillaries   e. Heart action — working phase
    ____ 6. Veins   f. Heart action — resting phase

Part 4.   *Column A*   *Column B*
    ____ 1. Digestion   a. Green liquid made in liver
    ____ 2. Saliva   b. Semi-solid waste material
    ____ 3. Peristalsis   c. Process of food breakdown
    ____ 4. Bile   d. Moistens food in the mouth
    ____ 5. Feces   e. Involuntary muscle contractions

Part 5.   *Column A*   *Column B*
    ____ 1. Gonads   a. Monthly release of ovum
    ____ 2. Semen   b. Breasts
    ____ 3. Ovulation   c. Another name for sex glands
    ____ 4. Mammary   d. Chemicals that regulate action of
            glands   glands and organs
    ____ 5. Fetus   e. Monthly release of uterine lining
    ____ 6. Menstruation   f. Fluid that carries sperm
    ____ 7. Hormones   g. Unborn baby

MULTIPLE CHOICE   Select the correct word or group of words in parentheses to complete each statement.

1. Tissue that covers the internal and external surface of the body is called (*epithelial, connective, muscle*) tissue.
2. The heart, brain, and kidneys are examples of (*tissues, organs, systems*).
3. The inner layer of the skin is called the (*epidermis, dermis*).
4. When the temperature outside the body is high, blood vessels in the skin will (*dilate, constrict*).
5. Bones that bear the weight of the body are called (*flat, irregular, long, short*) bones.
6. The point at which two or more bones meet is called a (*ligament, tendon, joint*).
7. (*Cartilage, Bone marrow*) cushions a joint to protect bone ends from rubbing together.
8. Another name for involuntary muscle is (*skeletal, striated, smooth*).
9. Muscles are connected to bones by (*ligaments, tendons, cartilage*).
10. A (*contraction, contracture*) occurs when a muscle shortens and causes a bone to move.

11. Reasoning, memory, vision, and hearing are controlled by the brain's (*brainstem, cerebral cortex, cerebellum*).
12. The opening in the middle of the iris of the eye is called the (*pupil, sclera, retina*).
13. The (*tympanic membrane, eustachian tube, auditory canal*) connects the middle ear with the throat.
14. The semicircular canals and the cochlea are found in the (*external, middle, inner*) ear.
15. Oxygen is picked up in the lungs by the (*red blood cells, white blood cells, platelets*).
16. The upper chambers of the heart are called (*ventricles, atria*).
17. The largest artery of the body is the (*vena cava, aorta*).
18. Venous blood is (*rich, poor*) in oxygen.
19. Another name for the voice box is the (*pharynx, larynx*).
20. The tiny one-celled air sacs in the lungs are called (*epiglottis, bronchus, alveoli*).
21. The esophagus moves the food down into the (*small intestine, gallbladder, stomach*).
22. Most food is absorbed from the (*small, large*) intestine.
23. Urine is stored in the (*kidney, bladder*) until the desire to urinate is felt.
24. The male hormone is called (*semen, testosterone, progesterone*).
25. The narrow section of the uterus is called the (*cervix, vagina, endometrium*).
26. The first day of the menstrual cycle begins with (*ovulation, menstruation*).
27. An example of an endocrine gland would be the (*pituitary, liver, uterus*).
28. Metabolism — the burning of food for heat and energy — is regulated by the (*parathyroid, thyroid, adrenal*) gland.
29. The amount of sugar in the blood is regulated by the (*thyroid gland, parathyroid gland, pancreas*).
30. The "master gland" is the (*parathyroid, pituitary, adrenal*) gland.

FILL IN

1. Name three functions of the skin.

    a. _____
    b. _____
    c. _____

UNDERSTANDING HOW THE BODY FUNCTIONS

21

2. Bones are grouped according to shape. Name the four types and give an example of each.

   a. _____ Example: _____
   b. _____ Example: _____
   c. _____ Example: _____
   d. _____ Example: _____

3. Muscles perform three important functions. They are:

   a. _____
   b. _____
   c. _____

4. The main parts of the brain are listed below. Write a function for each part.
   a. Cerebrum: _____
   b. Cerebellum: _____
   c. Brainstem: _____

5. Name the five major sense organs.

   a. _____ d. _____
   b. _____ e. _____
   c. _____

6. Write the function of each of the blood cells below.
   a. Red blood cells: _____
   b. White blood cells: _____
   c. Platelets: _____

7. Air travels through five main structures of the respiratory system to reach the lungs. List the structures in order.

   a. _____ d. _____
   b. _____ e. _____
   c. _____

8. Name the three parts of the small intestine.

   a. _____
   b. _____
   c. _____

9. Trace the path of urine by listing the structures of the urinary system in order.

   a. _____ c. _____
   b. _____ d. _____

10. Give a function for each reproductive structure listed below.
    a. Testes (testicles): _____
    b. Seminal vesicles: _____
    c. Prostate gland: _____
    d. Ovary: _____
    e. Fallopian tube: _____
    f. Uterus: _____
    g. Vagina: _____
    h. Mammary glands: _____

LABELING

In each of the figures that follow, identify the numbered parts on the lines provided.

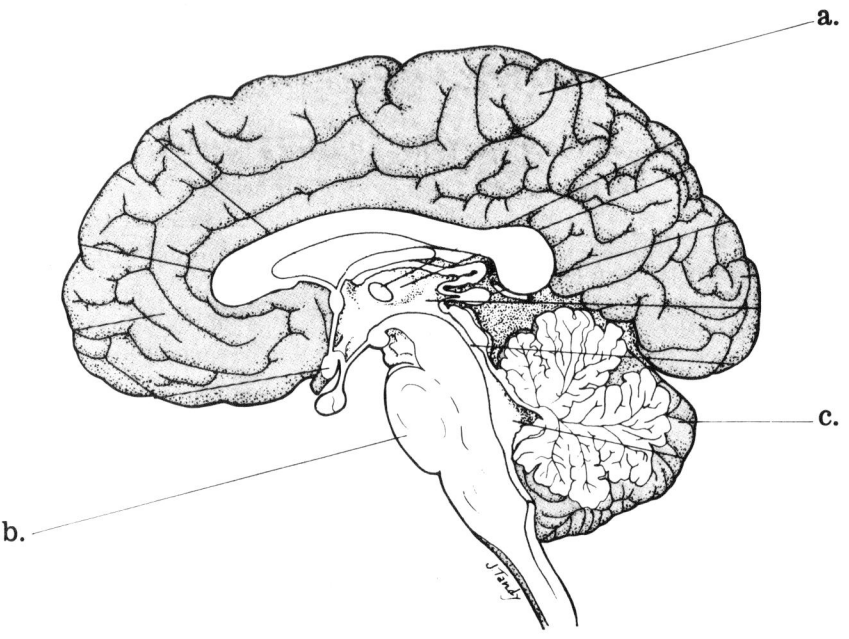

FIG. 6–1. The brain. (From Austrin, M. and Austrin, H.: Young's learning medical terminology step by step, ed. 6, St. Louis, 1987, The C. V. Mosby Co.)

a. _____
b. _____
c. _____

UNDERSTANDING HOW THE BODY FUNCTIONS 23

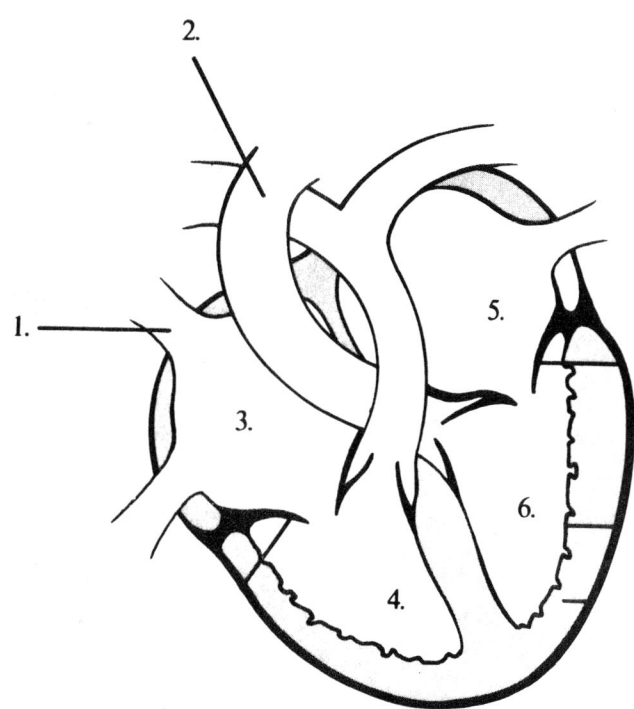

FIG. 6–2. The heart. (From Sorrentino, S. A.: Mosby's textbook for nursing assistants, ed. 2, St. Louis, 1987, The C. V. Mosby Co.)

1. _____
2. _____
3. _____
4. _____
5. _____
6. _____

In addition to identifying the parts of the heart, insert the arrows to show the flow of blood through the heart.

24 *MOSBY'S WORKBOOK FOR THE HOMEMAKER/HOME HEALTH AIDE*

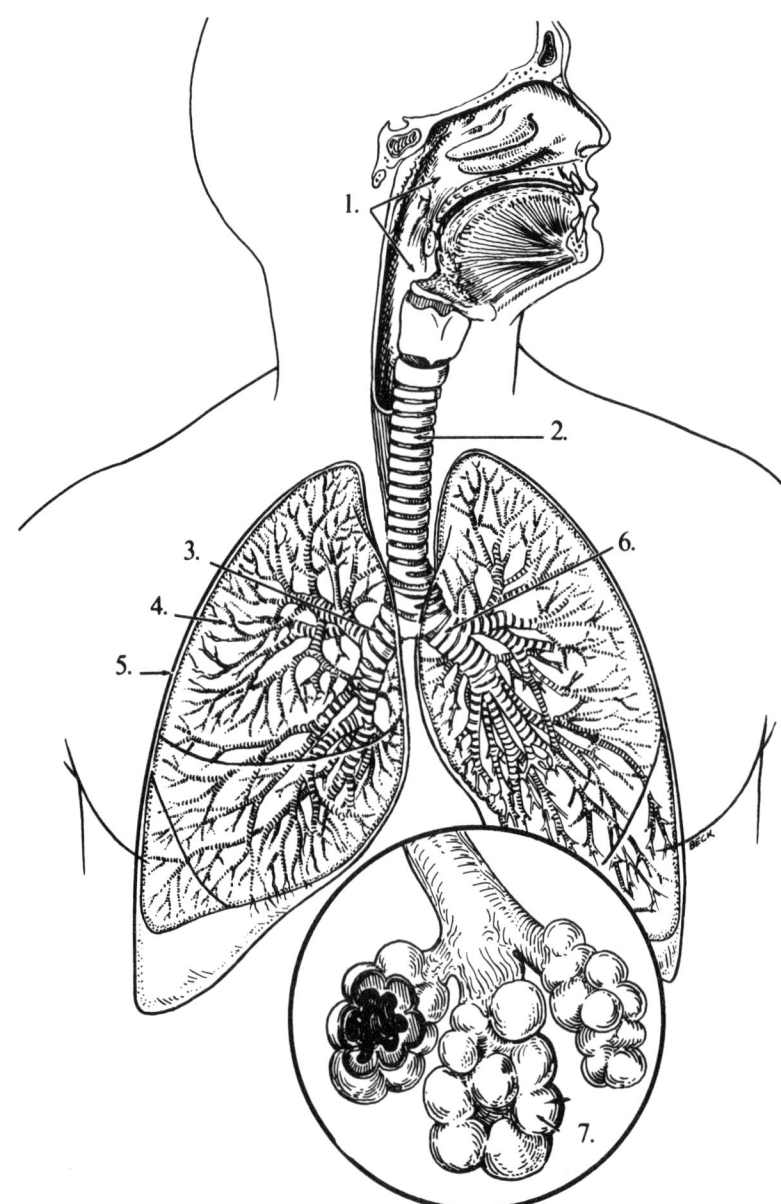

FIG. 6–3. The respiratory system. (Adapted from Anthony, C. P. and Thibodeau, G. A.: Textbook of Anatomy and Physiology, ed. 12, St. Louis, 1987, The C. V. Mosby Co.)

1. _____
2. _____
3. _____
4. _____
5. _____
6. _____
7. _____

UNDERSTANDING HOW THE BODY FUNCTIONS 25

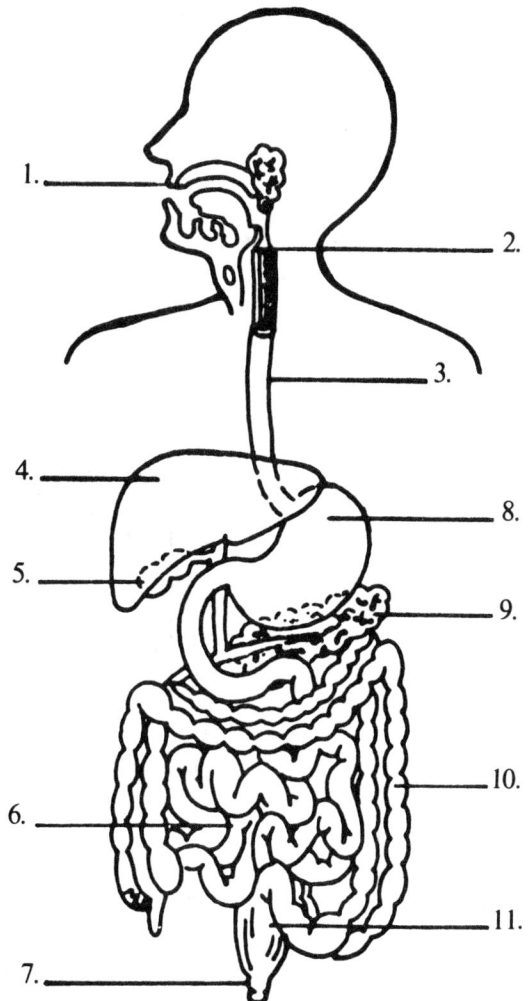

FIG. 6–4. The digestive system. (From Kelly, R. T.: Mosby's Workbook for Nursing Assistants, ed. 2, St. Louis, 1987, The C. V. Mosby Co.)

1. _____
2. _____
3. _____
4. _____
5. _____
6. _____
7. _____
8. _____
9. _____
10. _____
11. _____

26 *MOSBY'S WORKBOOK FOR THE HOMEMAKER/HOME HEALTH AIDE*

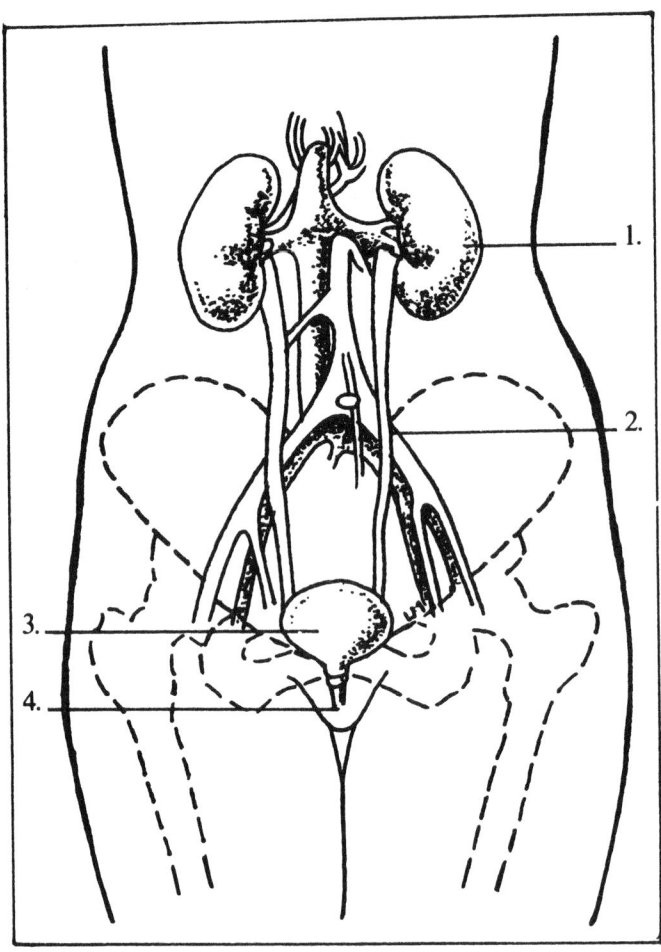

FIG. 6–5. The urinary system. (From Kelly, R. T.: Mosby's Workbook for Nursing Assistants, ed. 2, St. Louis, 1987, The C. V. Mosby Co.)

1. _____
2. _____
3. _____
4. _____

UNDERSTANDING HOW THE BODY FUNCTIONS 27

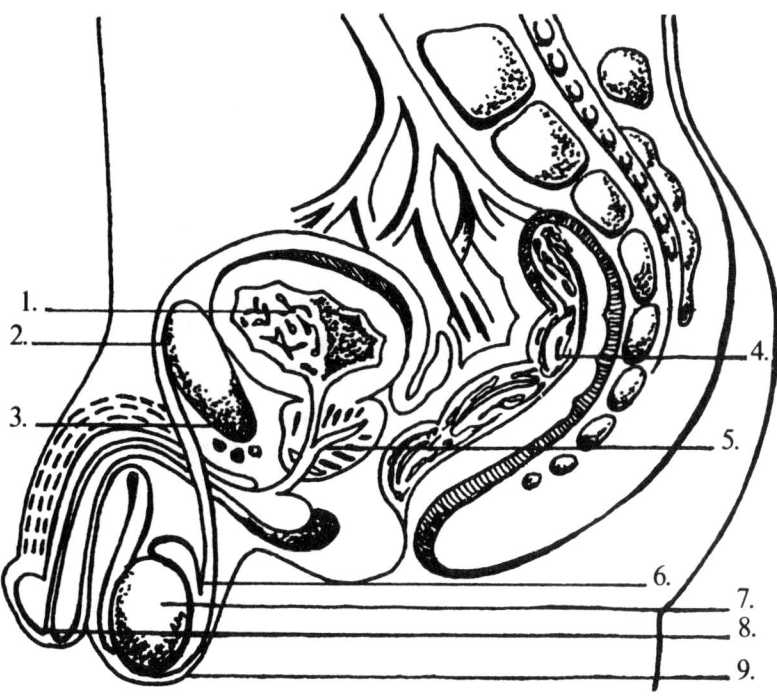

FIG. 6–6. The male reproductive system. (From Kelly, R. T.: Mosby's Workbook for Nursing Assistants, ed. 2, St. Louis, 1987, The C. V. Mosby Co.)

1. _____
2. _____
3. _____
4. _____
5. _____
6. _____
7. _____
8. _____
9. _____

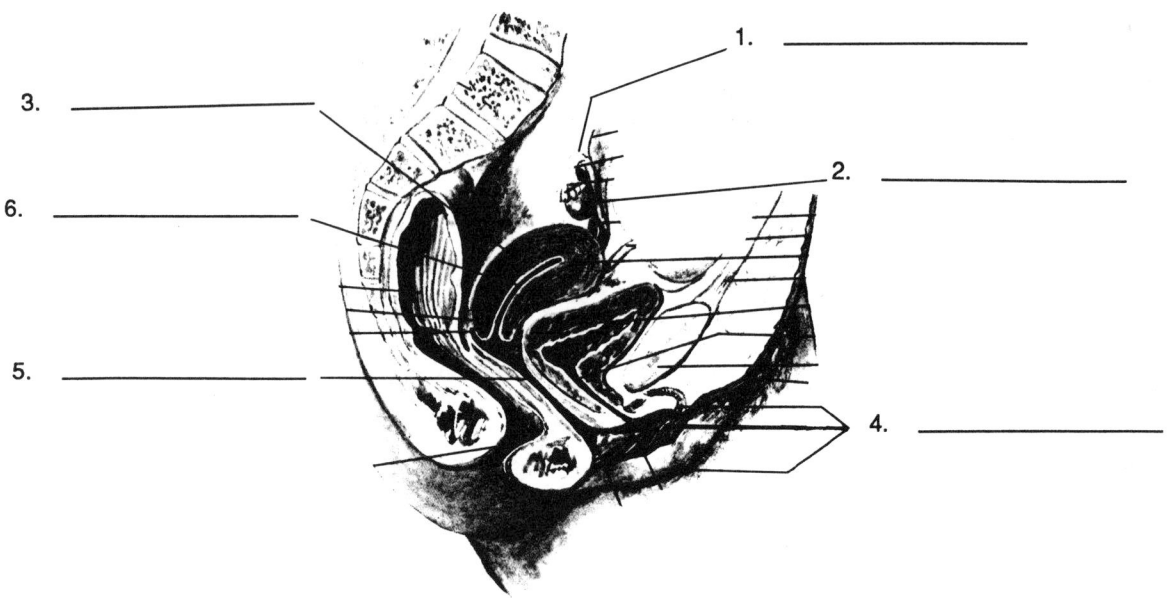

FIG. 6–7. The female reproductive system. (From Mosby's Medical and Nursing dictionary, ed. 2, St. Louis, 1986, The C. V. Mosby Co.)

1. _____
2. _____
3. _____
4. _____
5. _____
6. _____

WORD ASSOCIATION

Write the correct medical term for the common names of body parts and substances listed below.

	Common Name	Medical Term
1.	Bowel	_____
2.	Eardrum	_____
3.	Earwax	_____
4.	Throat	_____
5.	Voice box	_____
6.	White of the eye	_____
7.	Windpipe	_____
8.	Womb	_____

CHAPTER 7

Controlling Infection in the Home

TERMS TO KNOW Supply the correct term from the list to complete the sentences below.

asepsis clean technique contamination
disinfection infection medical asepsis
microorganism nonpathogen pathogen
sterile sterilization

1. The process by which all microorganisms are destroyed is called _____.
2. A _____ is a microorganism that can cause an infection.
3. _____ is the process by which an object or area becomes unclean.
4. The absence of pathogens is called _____.
5. Another term for medical asepsis is _____ _____.
6. A _____ is a small, living plant or animal that cannot be seen without a microscope.
7. The process by which pathogens are destroyed is known as _____.
8. The techniques and practices used to prevent the spread of pathogens is _____ _____.
9. _____ are microorganisms that do not generally cause infection.
10. When microorganisms invade and grow in the body and cause disease, the result is termed a/an _____.
11. An item is considered _____ if it is free of all microorganisms.

29

TRUE AND FALSE

Mark the statement "T" for true or "F" for false. Change the false statements to make them true.

_____ 1. Microorganisms need a dry area in order to live and grow.
_____ 2. Cold temperatures will kill microorganisms.
_____ 3. Light destroys microbes.
_____ 4. Medical asepsis is the same as disinfection.
_____ 5. If an item is sterile, it is free of all microorganisms, including pathogens.
_____ 6. In handwashing, sink faucets are considered clean.
_____ 7. Hold equipment and linens close to your uniform.
_____ 8. Always clean from the dirtiest to the cleanest areas.
_____ 9. Always wear disposable gloves and apron when you will be in contact with a client's body fluids.
_____ 10. Handwashing should last about one to two minutes using friction and rotating motions.
_____ 11. When cleaning equipment to be sterilized, rinse first in hot water to remove organic material.
_____ 12. Disinfection will destroy spores — the microorganisms that are protected by a hard shell.
_____ 13. A communicable disease is one that is contagious or easily spread.
_____ 14. Ideally, double bagging should be done by one person.
_____ 15. The most important infection control measure is handwashing.

CHECKING UP ON PROCEDURES

Number the following statements to show the correct order for performing these procedures.

Handwashing

_____ Clean under your fingernails with a nail brush.
_____ Apply soap to your hands.
_____ Turn off the faucet with paper towels.
_____ Wet your wrists and hands; keep hands lower than elbows.
_____ Dry your wrists and hands with paper towels.
_____ Wash each hand and wrist thoroughly.

Wet Heat Sterilization

_____ Bring the water to a boil.
_____ Place items in the pot.
_____ Wash your hands.
_____ Remove the items with tongs.

CONTROLLING INFECTION IN THE HOME

MULTIPLE CHOICE Select the correct word or group of words in parentheses to complete each statement.

1. Small items can be disinfected by placing them in boiling water for at least (*5, 10, 15*) minutes.
2. Microorganisms are destroyed by (*heat, cold*).
3. In wet heat sterilization, the water should boil for (*10, 20, 30*) minutes.
4. In isolation technique, the inside of the gown is considered (*clean, dirty*).
5. The correct order for removing isolation gear is (*gown-gloves-mask, mask-gloves-gown, gloves-gown-mask*).
6. Disinfection does not destroy (*pathogens, spores*).
7. Change your gown as soon as it becomes (*wet, contaminated*).
8. When removing your mask, touch only the (*ties, inside of the mask, outside of the mask*).
9. Gloves are easier to put on if your hands are (*wet, dry*).
10. Wash your hands (*after, before*) leaving the isolation area.

MATCHING Match the various types of isolation techniques on Column A with the correct definitions in Column B.

Column A

_____ 1. Drainage/secretion precautions
_____ 2. Respiratory isolation
_____ 3. Enteric precautions
_____ 4. Blood/body fluid precautions
_____ 5. Strict isolation

Column B

a. Used when body fluids are infected
b. Used to prevent the spread of pathogens through the air
c. Used to prevent the spread of pathogens found in wounds or wound drainage
d. Used to prevent the spread of pathogens through feces
e. Used when communicable diseases are spread by direct contact or through the air

LIST

1. Name six conditions that microorganisms must have to live and grow.

    a. _____
    b. _____
    c. _____
    d. _____
    e. _____
    f. _____

2. List at least six signs or symptoms of an infection.

    a. _____
    b. _____
    c. _____
    d. _____
    e. _____
    f. _____

3. Name three things needed for good handwashing.

    a. _____
    b. _____
    c. _____

CHAPTER 8

Safety

TRUE AND FALSE Mark the statement "T" for true or "F" for false. Change the false statements to make them true.

_____ 1. A client in a coma is completely unaware of his/her surroundings.
_____ 2. Burns are the most common accident in the home.
_____ 3. Most falls involving the elderly occur on stairs.
_____ 4. Wheels on beds and wheelchairs should not be locked when clients are being transferred.
_____ 5. Hot water heaters should be set at no more than 120° F for elderly clients.
_____ 6. To avoid electrical shocks, electrical equipment must be turned on before being unplugged.
_____ 7. When carrying a fire extinguisher, keep it upright.
_____ 8. When using a fire extinguisher, direct the hose at the top of the fire.
_____ 9. Do not allow strangers to use your telephone unless it is an emergency.
_____ 10. If you experience car trouble, stay in the car and keep the doors locked.

MULTIPLE CHOICE Select the correct word or group of words in parentheses to complete each statement.

1. Children and (*teenagers, young adults, the elderly*) have a special need to be protected from injury.
2. The client's bed should be in the (*low, high*) position except when giving bedside care.
3. For the client using oxygen, fabrics used for pajamas and clothing should be (*synthetic, wool, cotton*).
4. If a fire should occur in a client's home, (*close, open*) the doors as you leave the home.

5. Call bells should be placed on the client's (*good, weak, right*) side.
6. You should ask for a stranger's identification (*before, after*) you open the door.
7. If you are being followed in a car, drive to (*the nearest police or gas station, your home, the nearest driveway*).
8. When taking public transportation, it is a good idea to sit near (*an exit, the driver*).
9. When walking at night, walk in the street with the traffic (*to your back, facing you*).
10. If you suspect someone has broken into your home, (*go, do not go*) inside to check.

CHECKING UP ON PROCEDURES

Number the following statements to show the correct order for performing this procedure.

Using a Fire Extinguisher

_____ Remove the safety pin.
_____ Take the extinguisher to the fire.
_____ Direct the hose at the fire.
_____ Push the top handle down.
_____ Pull the fire alarm.

SAFE OR UNSAFE?

Mark the statement "S" if the action described is safe. Mark it "U" if it describes an unsafe action and tell why on the lines below.

_____ 1. You always keep the handles of pots and pans pointed toward the back of the stove.
_____ 2. You smell gas in your client's home. You open the windows for a while to air out the rooms.
_____ 3. The cord on your client's vacuum cleaner is frayed. You tape it with black electrical tape.
_____ 4. Your client is receiving oxygen. You remove the radio from his room, despite his objection.
_____ 5. You always have a list of fire and police emergency numbers in your purse when you are in a client's home.
_____ 6. You are feeding an infant in a high chair. The doorbell rings. You take the child with you to answer it.
_____ 7. Your client is elderly and has poor vision. You keep his medicines at the bedside table so they are easy for him to reach.

SAFETY 35

_____ 8. The tips on your client's walker are very worn. You remove them and replace them with new ones.

_____ 9. You receive a telephone call that is a "wrong number." You refuse to give the caller any information and ask what number he or she is trying to reach.

_____ 10. The light bulb in the client's hallway has burned out. You make a mental note of it and plan to replace it.

_____
_____
_____
_____
_____
_____
_____
_____

HIDDEN WORD SEARCH Write the correct word from the clues given on the broken lines. When you finish, the hidden word will appear by reading vertically.

1. Slick floors or a throw rug causes this   _ O _ _
2. Unconscious; not aware   _ O _ _ _
3. Choking or drowning can cause this   _ _ _ _ _ O _ _ _ _ _
4. Spark + oxygen + wood =   _ _ O _ _ _
5. Takes leaking electricity to earth   _ _ _ _ _ _ O _
6. "No smoking" where this is used   _ _ _ _ O _
7. Spilling hot liquids can cause these   _ _ _ O _
8. Caused by microorganisms spreading   _ _ _ _ O _ _ _
9. Childproof caps help prevent this   _ _ _ O _ _ _ _ _

CHAPTER 9

Home Maintenance

TERMS TO KNOW Match the terms listed in Column A with the correct definition from Column B.

Column A

_____ 1. All-purpose cleaner
_____ 2. Bleach
_____ 3. Cleanser
_____ 4. Detergent
_____ 5. Fabric softener
_____ 6. Soap
_____ 7. Specialty cleaner

Column B

a. A product used for laundry and dishwashing
b. A product used for certain surfaces and cleaning problems
c. Removes stains, brightens fabrics; disinfects
d. A product used for all types of cleaning
e. A product used for hard-to-clean surfaces such as sinks, tubs, toilets
f. Removes stiffness from fabrics
g. A product used for bathing, laundry, dishwashing

TRUE AND FALSE Mark the statement "T" for true or "F" for false. Change the false statements to make them true.

_____ 1. Light housekeeping duties include dusting, vacuuming, and washing floors.
_____ 2. A clean house is your first concern.
_____ 3. Sinks and tubs should be scrubbed with a powdered cleanser.
_____ 4. For very stubborn stains, mix several cleaning products to get the best result.

HOME MAINTENANCE

    _____ 5. Routine cleaning of the kitchen does not include waxing the floor.
    _____ 6. Refrigerate leftovers when they have cooled.
    _____ 7. The client's bed linens should be changed at least once a week.
    _____ 8. Washing laundry by hand cleans and disinfects better than by using a washing machine.
    _____ 9. Dry clothing completely before ironing.
    _____ 10. Stains should be treated as soon as possible for best results.

MULTIPLE CHOICE Select the correct word or group of words in parentheses to complete each statement.

1. To clean an oven you should use a/an (*all-purpose cleaner, specialty cleaner, powdered cleanser*).
2. If you splash a cleaning product into your eyes, rinse with running water for (*5, 10, 15*) minutes.
3. Leftover food must be used within (*1, 3, 5*) days.
4. Dishes are washed in hot, soapy water and rinsed in (*hot, warm, cool*) water.
5. When doing dishes, begin with the (*cleanest, dirtiest*) items first.
6. Wood and plastic items (*should, should not*) be placed in a dishwasher.
7. Dishes should be (*air, towel*) dried.
8. The client's bathroom should be cleaned (*daily, every other day, once a week*).
9. When soaking a stain from an article of clothing, use (*hot, warm, cold*) water.
10. Try (*bleach, prewash product, vinegar*) on stains first.

MATCHING Match the housekeeping tasks listed below with the letter that tells how often each task needs to be performed.

A = As needed   W = Weekly   D = Daily

    _____ 1. Change the linen on the client's bed.
    _____ 2. Change the water in flower vases.
    _____ 3. Clean the client's bedframe with a disinfectant.
    _____ 4. Pick up toys, newspapers, and magazines.
    _____ 5. Make the client's bed.

_____ 6. Empty ashtrays and wastebaskets.
_____ 7. Clean the client's bathroom.
_____ 8. Vacuum carpets and rugs.
_____ 9. Replace toilet paper and tissues.
_____ 10. Dust furniture in client's living area.
_____ 11. Empty garbage.
_____ 12. Put away clothes, dishes, and towels.
_____ 13. Wet mop uncarpeted floors.
_____ 14. Wash the client's water pitcher.
_____ 15. Wipe off the outside of kitchen cabinets.

CHAPTER 10

Body Mechanics

TERMS TO KNOW Match the terms listed in Column A in each section with the correct definition found in Column B.

Part 1.

Column A	Column B
____ 1. Base of support	a. Used to hold onto a client during transfer or when walking with the client
____ 2. Body mechanics	b. Rubbing of one surface against another
____ 3. Friction	c. Body alignment
____ 4. Posture	d. Area upon which an object rests
____ 5. Transfer belt	e. Using the body in an efficient and careful way

Part 2.

Column A	Column B
____ 1. Hemiparesis	a. Side of the body not affected by weakness or injury; strong side
____ 2. Hemiplegia	b. A person who is paralyzed from the waist down
____ 3. Involved side	c. A person who is paralyzed from the neck down
____ 4. Paralysis	d. A person who is paralyzed on one side of the body
____ 5. Paraplegic	e. Weakness on one side of the body
____ 6. Quadriplegic	f. Side of the body that does not function well; impaired side
____ 7. Uninvolved side	g. Loss of muscle function or sensation in a body part

LABELING　　Write the name of the basic position shown in each figure.

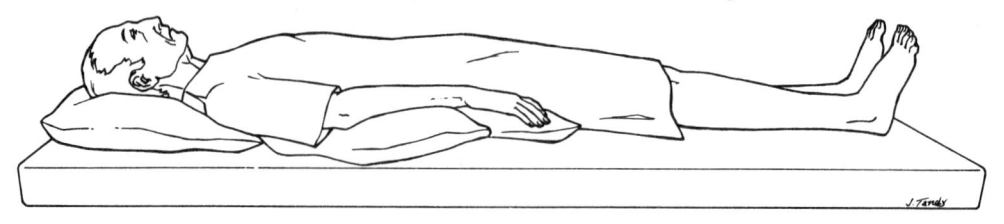

Fig. 10–1. _____

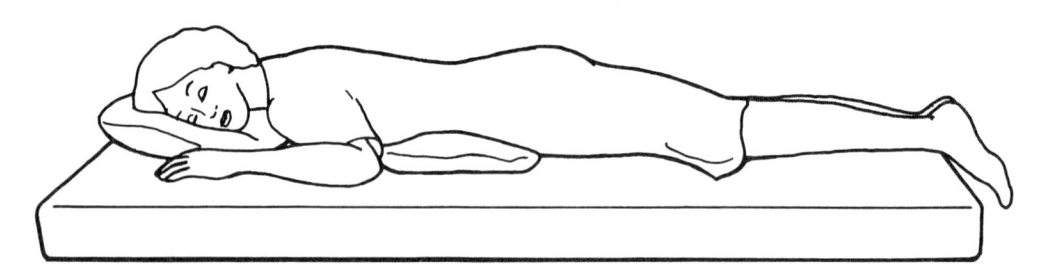

Fig. 10–2. _____

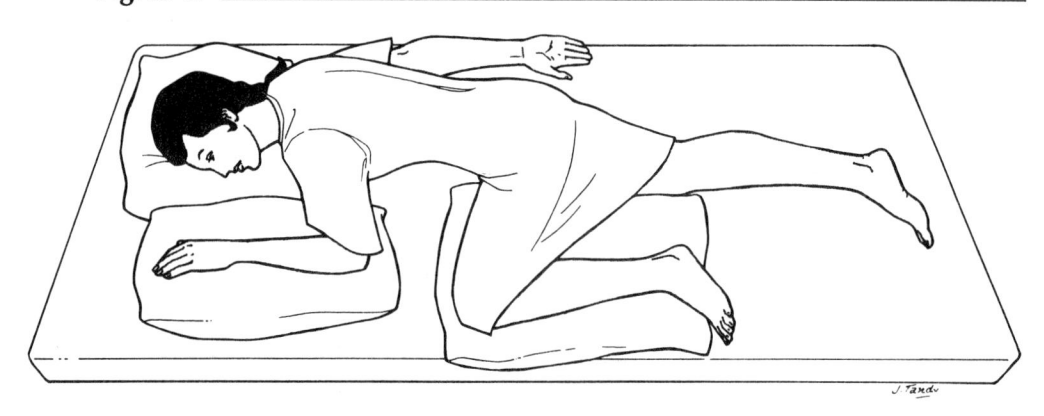

Fig. 10–3. _____

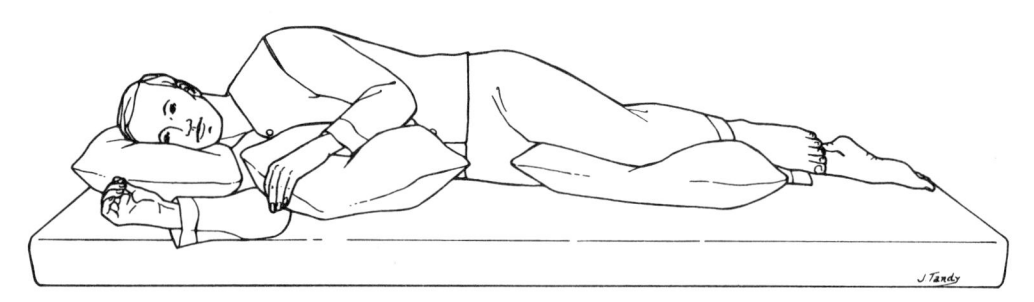

Fig. 10–4. _____

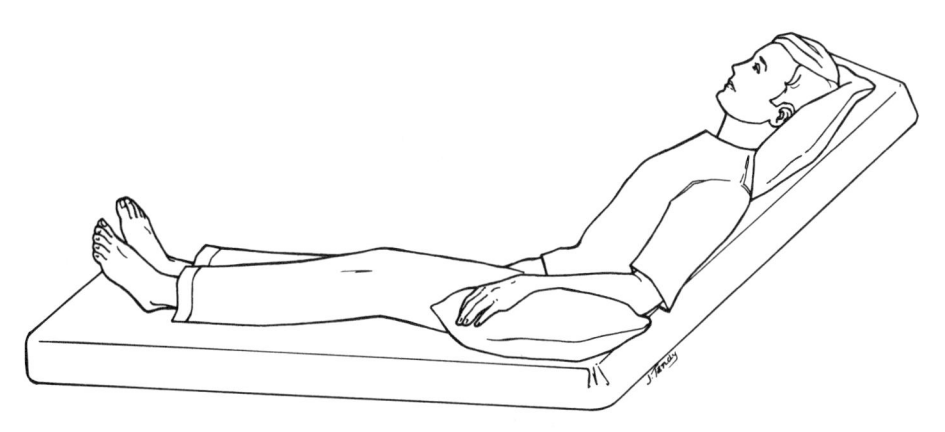

BODY MECHANICS   41

Fig. 10–5. _____

TRUE AND FALSE   Mark the statement "T" for true or "F" for false. Change the false statements to make them true.

_____ 1. The strongest and largest muscles are in the back.
_____ 2. Avoid lifting; push, pull, or slide instead.
_____ 3. The lateral position is the same as the dorsal recumbent position.
_____ 4. A client needs to be able to hold the upper body and head erect in order to sit in a chair.
_____ 5. A turning sheet helps reduce friction when moving a client in bed.
_____ 6. Allow a client to do as little as possible when transferring.
_____ 7. A transfer belt and a gait belt are the same device.
_____ 8. The buckle of the transfer belt should be positioned in the center of the abdomen.
_____ 9. When using a mechanical lift, have the client hold the swivel bar as you make the transfer.
_____ 10. You can do more damage if you try to stop a client from falling, than if you ease the client to the floor.

CHECKING UP ON PROCEDURES   Number the following statements to show the correct order for performing these procedures.

Moving Client Up in Bed with Client's Help

_____ Put the pillow under the client's head and shoulders. Ask the client to bend the knees.
_____ Move the client to the head of the bed shifting your body weight.

_____ Place one arm under the shoulders and the other under the client's knees.
_____ Ask the client to push with the hands and feet on a count of three.

Moving a Client to the Side of the Bed

_____ Place one arm under the client's waist, the other under the thighs.
_____ Place one arm under the client's thighs and the other under the calves. Move the legs and feet toward you.
_____ Move the upper part of the client's body toward you.
_____ Place one arm under the client's neck and shoulders, the other under the midback.
_____ Move the lower part of the client's body toward you.

Transferring the Client to a Chair/Wheelchair

_____ Brace your knees against the client's knees; block his or her feet with your feet.
_____ Turn the client so he or she can grasp the far arm of the chair; continue to turn to reach the other armrest.
_____ Help the client put on a robe.
_____ Pull the client up into a standing position.
_____ Stand in front of the client.
_____ Lower the client into the chair.

Protecting the Client During a Fall

_____ Move your leg so that the client's buttocks rest on your leg.
_____ Call for help if someone else is in the home.
_____ Check the client for injuries.
_____ Call your supervisor.
_____ Bring the client close to your body as quickly as possible.
_____ Lower the client to the floor by allowing him or her to slide down your leg.

MULTIPLE CHOICE Select the correct word or group of words in parentheses to complete each statement.

1. A (*wide, narrow*) base of support makes you feel more balanced and stable.
2. Lift and carry objects with your palms (*up, down*) in order to use the larger muscles of your upper arm.

3. In Fowler's position, the head of the bed is (*flat, raised slightly, 45 to 60 degrees*).
4. When positioned in a chair, the back of the client's knees and calves should be (*touching, slightly away from*) the edge of the seat.
5. (*Rolling, sliding*) clients helps reduce friction when moving in bed.
6. If moving the client causes pain, (*quickly finish the move, stop immediately*).
7. Apply a transfer belt (*over, under*) the client's clothing.
8. Transfer a client from his or her (*strong, weak*) side.
9. If a client is unconscious after a fall, (*lift the client back into bed with assistance, call an ambulance.*)
10. The vinyl seats and backs on wheelchairs tend to make a client feel (*cold, warm*).

CHAPTER 11
Activity

TERMS TO KNOW Using the list below, write the term on the line with the correct definition.

activities of daily living   embolus   atrophy
contracture   prosthesis   footdrop
plantar flexion   thrombus   range of motion
rehabilitation

_____ 1. An artificial replacement for a missing body part
_____ 2. A blood clot that travels through blood vessels
_____ 3. Another term for plantar flexion
_____ 4. The things we do every day
_____ 5. A decrease in size or a wasting away of tissue
_____ 6. Movement of a joint to the extent possible without causing pain
_____ 7. A blood clot
_____ 8. The process of restoring the disabled person to the highest level of functioning
_____ 9. Abnormal shortening of a muscle
_____ 10. Bending of the foot

TRUE AND FALSE Mark the statement "T" for true or "F" for false. Change the false statements to make them true.

_____ 1. A transfer (gait) belt should be used when ambulating a weak or unsteady client.

_____ 2. When you ambulate a client, be sure to walk at his or her strong side.

_____ 3. The home health aide will teach the client to use walking aids, such as crutches.

ACTIVITY 45

_____ 4. Baskets and pouches may not be attached to a walker.
_____ 5. A walker gives a client more support than a cane.
_____ 6. A footboard is the same as a bed cradle.
_____ 7. Trochanter rolls prevent the hips and legs from turning outward.
_____ 8. A contracture is a permanent deformity of a muscle.
_____ 9. When the client does range of motion (ROM) exercises without help it is called active ROM.
_____ 10. Usually, ROM exercises are repeated two to three times per joint.
_____ 11. In ROM, never force a joint to the point of pain.

MULTIPLE CHOICE Select the correct word or group of words in parentheses to complete each statement.

1. The client using crutches should wear (*loose, well-fitting*) clothing.
2. A single-tipped cane is held on the client's (*strong, weak*) side.
3. Three and four-point canes are usually held on the client's (*strong, weak*) side.
4. Muscle atrophy is a/an (*increase, decrease*) in the size of a muscle.
5. Handrolls can be made by using (*folded blankets, pillows, rolled washcloths*).
6. When another person moves the joints through ROM exercises, it is called (*active, passive, active-assistive*).
7. If possible, position the client in the (*supine, prone, side-lying*) position for ROM exercises.
8. ROM exercises usually begin with the (*hands, feet, neck*).
9. An example of a prosthesis is a/an (*brace, artificial eye, plate guard*).
10. In the rehabilitation process, it is important to concentrate on the person's (*abilities, disabilities*).

CHECKING UP ON PROCEDURES Number the following statements to show the correct order for performing this procedure.

Helping the Client Walk

_____ Help the client put on a robe.
_____ Help the client put on shoes.
_____ Help the client stand.
_____ Help the client sit on the side of the bed.
_____ Apply the transfer belt.
_____ Give the client any walking aid used.

MATCHING

Match the movement in Column A with the correct description in Column B.

	Column A		Column B
_____	1. Abduction	a.	Turning downward
_____	2. Adduction	b.	Turning the joint
_____	3. Extension	c.	Excessive straightening of a body part
_____	4. Flexion	d.	Moving away from the body
_____	5. Hyperextension	e.	Straightening a body part
_____	6. Dorsiflexion	f.	Turning upward
_____	7. Rotation	g.	Moving toward the body
_____	8. Internal rotation	h.	Bending a body part
_____	9. External rotation	i.	Turning a joint inward
_____	10. Pronation	j.	Bending backward
_____	11. Supination	k.	Turning a joint outward

ACTIVITY

CROSSWORD PUZZLE

Complete the crossword puzzle using the clues below.

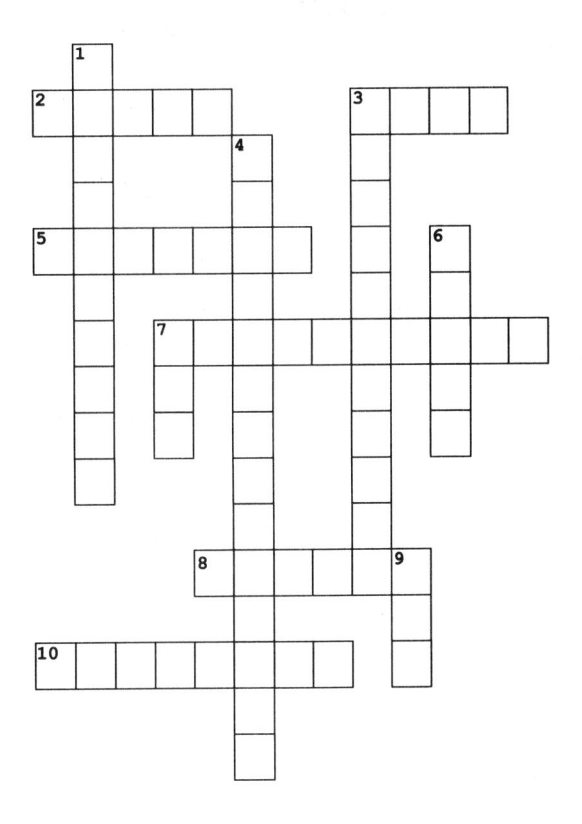

Across:
2. Used to support a weak body part or to prevent movement or deformity
3. Single-tipped or three- and four-point type
5. Wasting away of tissue
7. Act of walking
8. A common four-point walking aid
10. Bedsores

Down:
1. Artificial body part
3. Abnormal shortening of a muscle
4. Process of restoring an individual to the highest level of functioning
6. Point at which two or more bones come together
7. Activities of daily living
9. Range of motion

CHAPTER 12

Bedmaking

TERMS TO KNOW Supply the correct term from the list to complete the sentences below.

closed bed   drawsheet   Fowler's
mitered corner   occupied bed   open bed
plastic drawsheet   semi-Fowler's   Trendelenburg's

1. Tucking linens under the mattress in such a way as to keep the linens straight and smooth is known as a _____ _____.
2. When the head of the bed is lowered and the foot is raised, the bed is said to be in _____ position.
3. A/an _____ _____ is a bed that is made with the client remaining in it.
4. A _____ is a sheet placed over the middle of the bottom sheet that can be used to turn and move clients in bed.
5. When a bed is not going to be used for most of the day, a _____ _____ is made.
6. When the top linens are folded back so that the client can get into bed easily, the bed is known as a/an _____ _____.
7. _____ position is a semisitting position with the head of the bed elevated 45 to 60 degrees.
8. In order to keep the mattress and bottom linens clean and dry, a _____ _____ is used in bedmaking.
9. _____ position means having the head of the bed raised 45 degrees, while the knee portion may or may not be raised (depending on agency policy).

TRUE AND FALSE Mark the statement "T" for true or "F" for false. Change the false statements to make them true.

_____ 1. Beds should be in the high position only when giving client care.

_____ 2. Hand cranks on manually operated hospital beds should be in the up position when not in use.

BEDMAKING

49

_____ 3. The knee portion of a bed is raised 15 degrees when a bed is placed in Trendelenburg's position.

_____ 4. The thermostat on a water bed needs to be checked every day to ensure client comfort.

_____ 5. Dirty linen should be placed on the floor.

_____ 6. A plastic drawsheet must be used with a cotton drawsheet.

_____ 7. A top sheet may be reused as a bottom sheet if there is a shortage of linen.

_____ 8. Make as much of one side of the bed as possible before going to the other side.

_____ 9. A plastic drawsheet should be placed about 24 inches from the top of the mattress.

_____ 10. Bed linens should be changed as soon as they become wet, soiled, or damp.

LABELING

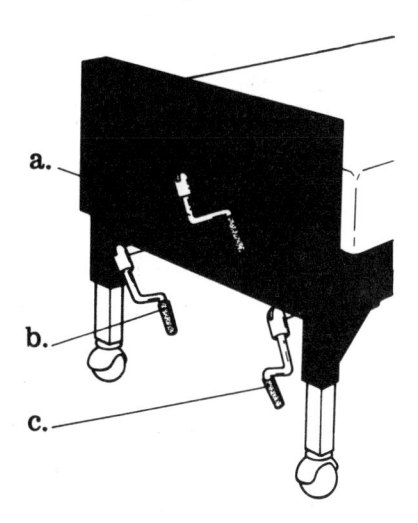

FIG. 12–1. (From Sorrentino, S. A.: Mosby's Textbook for Nursing Assistants, ed. 2, St. Louis, 1987, The C. V. Mosby Co.)

1. Figure 12–1 shows the hand cranks of the manually operated hospital bed. Tell what each crank does on the lines below.

   a. _____
   b. _____
   c. _____

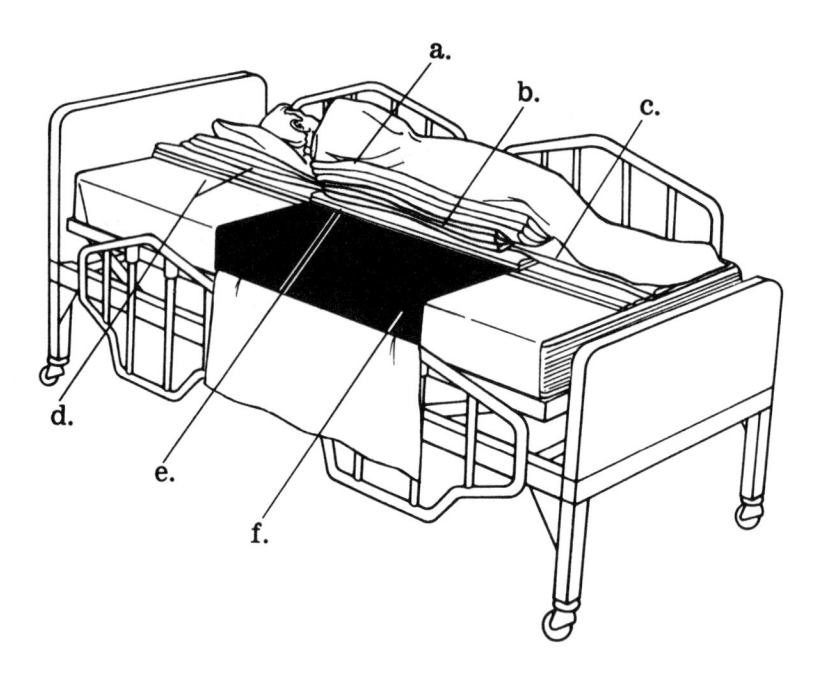

FIG. 12-2. (From Sorrentino, S. A.: Mosby's Textbook for Nursing Assistants, ed. 2, St. Louis, 1987, The C. V. Mosby Co.)

2. Name each piece of linen as it appears on the bed in Figure 12-2.

a. _____
b. _____
c. _____
d. _____
e. _____
f. _____

MULTIPLE CHOICE

Select the correct word or group of words in parentheses to complete each statement.

1. The client's bed needs to be stripped and allowed to air out at least (*once a day, once a week*).
2. Always hold linens (*away from, next to*) your body and uniform.
3. When placing a flat bottom sheet on the client's bed, the hem stitching should be (*toward, away from*) the mattress pad.
4. The (*cotton drawsheet, plastic drawsheet, pillowcase*) can be reused if it is not soiled, wet, or very wrinkled.
5. Instead of plastic drawsheets, some clients may use (*mattress pads, disposable bed protectors*) to keep the bottom linen and mattress clean and dry.

6. Torn bed linen should be (*pinned together, discarded, mended*).
7. When collecting linens, the last item should be the (*mattress pad, top sheet, pillowcase*).
8. In bedmaking, the top sheet, blanket, and bedspread should (*not be tucked in, be tucked in together, be tucked in separately*) at the foot of the bed.
9. The pillow should be placed on the bed so that the open end is (*away from, facing*) the door.
10. Offer the client the bedpan or urinal (*before, after*) making the occupied bed.

CHAPTER 13

Vital Signs

TERMS TO KNOW Match the terms listed in Column A with the correct definition from Column B.

Column A

____ 1. Blood pressure
____ 2. Diastolic pressure
____ 3. Pulse
____ 4. Pulse deficit
____ 5. Respiration
____ 6. Sphygmomanometer
____ 7. Stethoscope
____ 8. Systolic pressure
____ 9. Temperature
____ 10. Vital signs

Column B

a. Pressure in the arteries when the heart is contracting
b. Instrument used to measure blood pressure
c. Temperature, pulse, respirations, and blood pressure
d. Amount of heat in the body
e. Amount of force exerted against the walls of an artery by the blood
f. The beat of the heart felt at an artery
g. Breathing air in and out of the lungs
h. Pressure in the arteries when the heart is relaxing
i. Instrument used to listen to the heart and other body sounds
j. Difference between apical and radial pulse rates

TRUE AND FALSE Mark the statement "T" for true or "F" for false. Change the false statements to make them true.

____ 1. Measure vital signs on all clients four times a day.
____ 2. You do not need to record the vital signs if they are within normal range.

VITAL SIGNS

___ 3. To shake down a thermometer, hold it securely at the stem, flex and snap your wrist until the mercury is shaken down.

___ 4. Rectal temperatures should not be taken on unconscious clients.

___ 5. The normal range of an adult pulse rate is 80 to 120 beats per minute.

___ 6. When listening to the heartbeat, each "lub-dub" is counted as one beat.

___ 7. Blood pressure cuffs may be applied over clothing.

___ 8. When taking a blood pressure, the client's arm should be positioned above the level of the heart with the palms up.

___ 9. An infant can be positioned on his or her back with the knees flexed toward the abdomen for a rectal temperature.

___ 10. The respiratory pattern of an infant is often irregular.

MULTIPLE CHOICE Select the correct word or group of words in parentheses to complete each statement.

1. A client's vital signs are usually lower in the (*morning, afternoon, night*).
2. When one vital sign changes, the other signs usually (*stay the same, change*).
3. Body heat is produced by the muscles (*only during exercise, constantly*).
4. Normal body temperature is (*99.7° F, 97.6° F, 98.6° F*) when measured orally.
5. (*Axillary, Rectal*) temperatures are one Fahrenheit degree lower than oral temperatures.
6. The tip of a glass thermometer used for rectal temperatures is (*long and slender, round and stubby*) and may be colored (*red, blue*).
7. When cleaning a glass thermometer, wipe from the (*stem to the bulb, bulb to the stem*).
8. The glass thermometer should be washed in (*hot, warm, cold*) soapy water.
9. When the client has been drinking fluids, wait (*5, 15, 30*) minutes before taking an oral temperature.
10. (*Oral, Rectal, Axillary*) temperatures are the least accurate.
11. A stethoscope is needed to take a/an (*apical, radial, carotid*) pulse.
12. If a pulse is irregular, it must be counted for (*30 seconds, 1 minute*).
13. The apical pulse is located on the (*left, right*) side of the chest.

14. Stethoscopes are cleaned before and after each use with (*soap and water, alcohol wipes*).
15. (*Tell, Do not tell*) the client that the respiratory rate is being counted.
16. Blood pressure above the normal range is known as (*hypertension, hypotension*).
17. The sphygmomanometer that has a round dial and a needle that points to the gauge is a/an (*aneroid, mercury, electronic*) type.
18. A blood pressure cuff is the correct size if it covers (*all, one-half, two-thirds*) of the upper arm.
19. The first number recorded on a blood pressure reading is the (*diastolic, systolic*) pressure.
20. Apical pulses are taken on infants and children up to age (*2, 3, 5*).

CHECKING UP ON PROCEDURES

Number the following statements to show the correct order for performing these procedures.

Measuring a Rectal Temperature

_____ Put on disposable gloves. Wipe the anal area to remove any lubricant or feces.
_____ Position the client in Sims' position.
_____ Read the thermometer.
_____ Wipe the thermometer with toilet tissue.
_____ Put a small amount of lubricant on a tissue and lubricate the bulb end of the thermometer.
_____ Insert the bulb end of the thermometer one inch into the rectum.

Taking a Radial Pulse

_____ Note if the pulse is strong or weak, regular or irregular.
_____ Locate the radial pulse.
_____ Record the pulse on paper.
_____ Have the client rest for 5 to 10 minutes.
_____ Have the client sit or lie down.
_____ Count the pulse for 30 seconds.

Taking an Apical Pulse

_____ Expose the nipple area of the left chest.
_____ Position the client in a lying or sitting position.
_____ Locate the apical pulse.
_____ Count the pulse for one full minute.
_____ Warm the diaphragm of the stethoscope in your palm.

VITAL SIGNS 55

Taking a Blood Pressure

_____ Place the diaphragm of the stethoscope over the brachial artery.
_____ Inflate the cuff 30 mm Hg beyond the point where you last felt the pulse. Deflate the cuff at an even rate.
_____ Place the arrow marking on the cuff over the brachial artery.
_____ Find the radial artery and inflate the cuff.
_____ Note the point where you hear the first sound and where the sound disappears.
_____ Deflate the cuff completely.

READING THERMOMETERS Read the thermometers, and write the answers on the lines provided below the figures. Convert your answers to Centigrade equivalents.

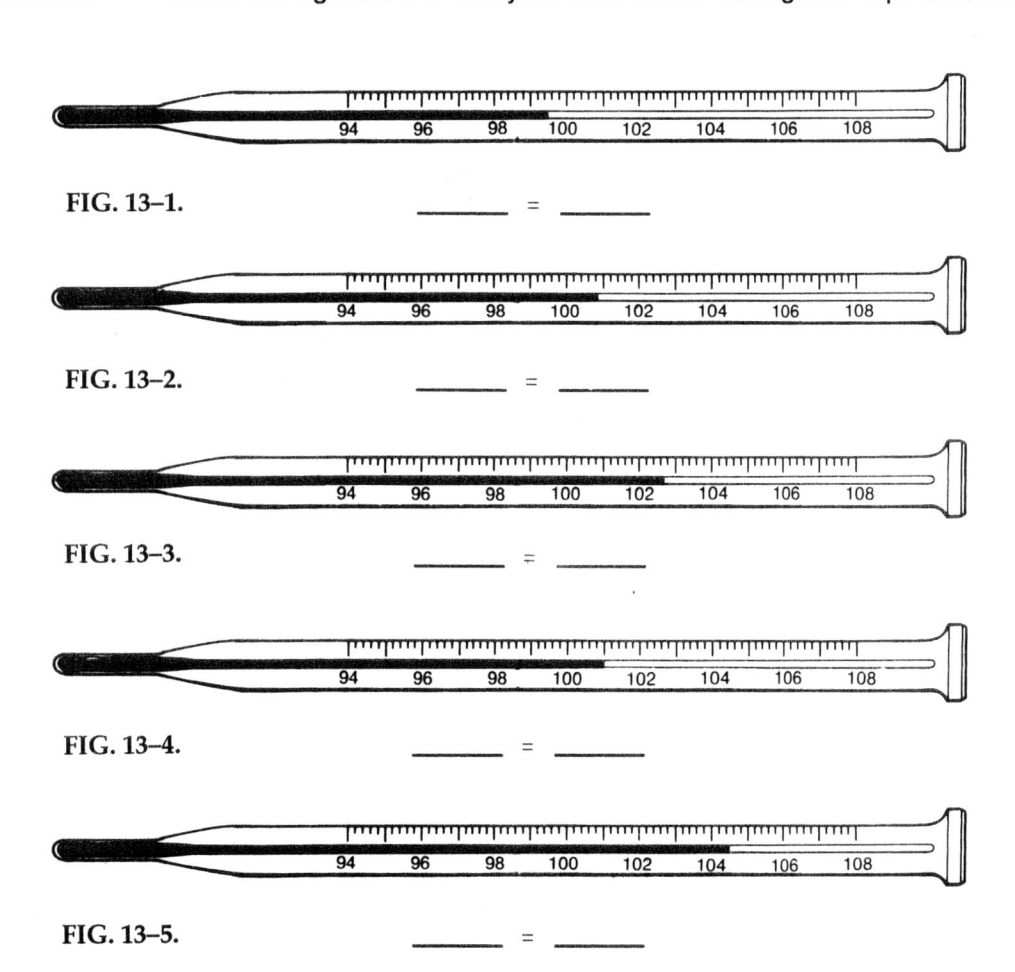

FIG. 13–1.   _____ = _____

FIG. 13–2.   _____ = _____

FIG. 13–3.   _____ = _____

FIG. 13–4.   _____ = _____

FIG. 13–5.   _____ = _____

CHARTING VITAL SIGNS

The following is an example of a graphic sheet typically used to record client's vital signs. Use the form below to record the following vital signs:

3/25/89 TPR 98.6 - 78 - 16 BP 138/84
3/26/89 TPR 97.4 - 72 - 16 BP 126/80
3/27/89 TPR 97.8 - 80 - 20 BP 122/70
3/28/89 TPR 98.4 - 76 - 14 BP 130/80
3/29/89 TPR 99.8 - 88 - 20 BP 136/88

VITAL SIGNS

LIST

1. Vital signs may need to be taken at times other than when instructed. List five occasions or reasons for taking a client's vital signs.

    a. _____
    b. _____
    c. _____
    d. _____
    e. _____

2. Blood pressure is affected by many factors. List five of those factors below.

    a. _____
    b. _____
    c. _____
    d. _____
    e. _____

3. List the normal ranges of body temperature for adults.

    a. Oral: _____
    b. Rectal: _____
    c. Axillary: _____

4. Name five sites on the body where the pulse can be taken.

    a. _____
    b. _____
    c. _____
    d. _____
    e. _____

CROSSWORD PUZZLE

Complete the crossword puzzle using the clues below.

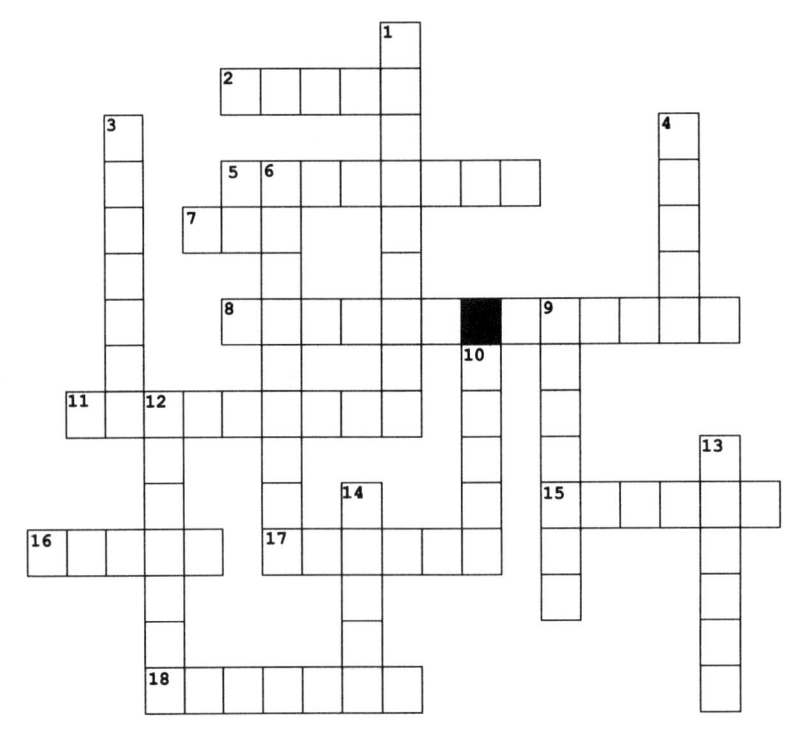

Across:
2. Elevated temperature
5. Strong or full pulse
7. Abbreviation for temperature, pulse, and respiration
8. Breathing pattern in which respirations gradually increase in rate and depth and then become shallow and slow
11. Rapid breathing
15. Heartbeat heard over the heart
16. Beat of the heart felt at an artery
17. Underarm
18. Period of heart muscle contraction

Down:
1. Slow breathing
3. Difficult, labored, or painful breathing
4. Strength of a heartbeat
5. Abbreviation for blood pressure
6. Needing to sit in order to breathe comfortably
9. Weak, feeble pulse
10. Lack of or absence of breathing
12. Centigrade
13. Common site for pulse measurement, at the wrist
14. TPR and BP are signs

CHAPTER 14

Personal Care

TERMS TO KNOW Using the list below, write the term on the line with the correct definition.

antiperspirant   aspiration   decubitus ulcer
deodorant   perineal care

_____ 1. An area where the skin and underlying tissues are eroded due to a lack of blood flow; bedsore

_____ 2. A preparation that masks and controls body odors

_____ 3. A skin care product that reduces the amount of perspiration

_____ 4. Cleansing the genital and anal areas of the body

_____ 5. The breathing of fluid or an object into the lungs

TRUE AND FALSE Mark the statement "T" for true or "F" for false. Change the false statements to make them true.

_____ 1. The nurse decides how much assistance a client needs with hygiene practices.

_____ 2. The client should receive as much assistance as possible with personal care needs.

_____ 3. You should choose the time and order of each personal care activity.

_____ 4. It is not necessary to wear gloves when giving oral hygiene.

_____ 5. Clients with fevers will need oral hygiene more frequently.

_____ 6. Clients should not practice oral hygiene while receiving oxygen.

_____ 7. Flossing the teeth is usually done after brushing.

_____ 8. Always assume that an unconscious client can hear.
_____ 9. Cold water causes dentures to warp.
_____ 10. You may change the bathing methods if a client requests it.
_____ 11. Soap is not needed for every bath.
_____ 12. When cleaning the eyes, use water only and wipe from the inner to the outer aspect.
_____ 13. Change the bath water twice during the bed bath.
_____ 14. Clients with IVs are allowed to shower.
_____ 15. Always leave the room while the client is in the shower.
_____ 16. Lotion is used during the back massage to reduce friction.
_____ 17. Pericare involves cleaning the face, hands, axillae, and genital areas.
_____ 18. You may braid the client's hair if she requests it.
_____ 19. Soak the feet before cutting the toenails.
_____ 20. The first sign of a decubitus ulcer is an open sore that is red and painful.
_____ 21. Preventing a decubitus ulcer is easier than healing one.
_____ 22. Keeping skin in contact with skin on the body helps reduce moisture and friction.
_____ 23. Massage reddened or pale pressure points with an up and down motion using lotion.
_____ 24. Clients should be encouraged to wear regular clothes during the day.
_____ 25. The side of the body receiving the IV should be dressed first.

MULTIPLE CHOICE Select the correct word or group of words in parentheses to complete each statement.

1. Clients who need help with most personal care activities such as bathing and dressing would be considered (*minimal, moderate, maximum*) assistance.
2. Toothbrushes for oral hygiene should have (*soft, hard*) bristles.
3. If a client is unable to sit up for oral hygiene, the (*supine, prone, side-lying*) position should be used instead.
4. Your client prefers to floss his or her teeth once a day. The best time is (*before breakfast, after lunch, at bedtime*).

5. When flossing the client's teeth, use a piece of floss about (*12, 18, 24*) inches long.
6. You would begin to floss the client's teeth at the (*lower right side, upper right side, center*) of the mouth.
7. The mouth of the unconscious client will need to be kept open for oral hygiene by using (*a padded tongue blade, your fingers*).
8. The outer surfaces of the front teeth should be brushed using a/an (*back-and-forth, up-and-down, circular*) motion.
9. Dentures that are not being worn should be kept in a (*dry plastic container, container filled with cool water, sealed plastic bag*).
10. A skin care product that absorbs moisture and prevents friction is (*soap, bath oil, powder*).
11. The temperature of the water for a bed bath should be (*105° F, 110 to 115° F, 115 to 120° F*).
12. When giving a bed bath, wash the arm (*nearest, farthest*) from you first.
13. The last area to be washed during a bed bath is the (*feet, back, perineum*).
14. The back is massaged (*before, during, after*) the bed bath.
15. A tub bath should last no longer than (*10, 20, 30*) minutes.
16. Water for a tub bath should be (*98.6, 105, 115*) degrees Fahrenheit.
17. A back massage should last (*1 to 3, 4 to 6, 8 to 10*) minutes.
18. In perineal care, clean the (*urethral, anal*) area last.
19. Clients confined to bed need to be repositioned every (*2, 4, 8*) hours.
20. When removing a client's clothing, start on the (*stronger, weaker*) side.

MATCHING

Match the decubitus care items in Column A with the correct descriptions in Column B.

Column A

_____ 1. Sheepskin
_____ 2. Bed cradles
_____ 3. Heel and elbow protectors
_____ 4. Flotation pads
_____ 5. Egg crate mattress
_____ 6. Water beds
_____ 7. Air mattress

Column B

a. Foam pads with peaks to distribute the client's weight more evenly; small pockets let the air circulate underneath
b. Made of foam rubber or sheepskin, they are shaped to provide extra padding and prevent friction between the linens and bony areas

c. Available in various sizes, allows air to circulate between the fur to help keep the skin dry and reduces friction between the skin and bottom sheet
d. Lets the client float on top of mattress; body weight is distributed along the entire length of the body, so pressure on bony points is avoided
e. Cushion made of a gel-like substance encased in heavy plastic, used for chairs and wheelchairs; expensive
f. Metal frames placed on beds to keep the weight of the top linen off the client's legs and feet
g. Made of plastic; placed on a regular mattress and covered with a sheet; body weight is distributed evenly

CHECKING UP ON PROCEDURES

Number the following statements to show the correct order for performing these procedures.

Providing Mouth Care for an Unconscious Client

_____ Separate the upper and lower teeth with the padded tongue blade.
_____ Place the emesis basin or bowl under his or her chin.
_____ Put on the gloves.
_____ Clean the mouth using swabs moistened with mouthwash or other solution.
_____ Place the towel under the client's face.
_____ Position the client on the side toward you with the head well turned.

Denture Care

_____ Apply some denture cleaner or toothpaste to the brush.
_____ Place dentures in the denture cup and fill with cool water.
_____ Line the sink with a towel, and fill the sink half full with water.
_____ Rinse each denture under warm, running water.
_____ Brush the dentures and rinse.

Giving a Partial Bath

_____ Help the client undress.
_____ Give a back massage.
_____ Have the client wash body parts that he or she can easily reach.
_____ Change the bath water.
_____ Position the client so he or she can bathe comfortably.
_____ Ask the client what was washed and wash the remaining areas.

PERSONAL CARE 63

Giving a Back Massage

_____ Position the client in the prone or side-lying position.
_____ Massage bony areas.
_____ Expose the back, shoulders, upper arms, and buttocks.
_____ Stroke upward from the buttocks to the shoulders, downward over the upper arms, and then reverse.
_____ Warm your hands and the lotion.
_____ Knead by grasping tissue between the thumb and fingers.

LIST

1. Bathing a client gives an excellent opportunity to observe the skin. List five observations that need to be reported to the nurse.

   a. _____
   b. _____
   c. _____
   d. _____
   e. _____

2. Name five types of clients that are at risk of developing decubitus ulcers.

   a. _____
   b. _____
   c. _____
   d. _____
   e. _____

CHAPTER 15

Elimination

TERMS TO KNOW Supply the correct term from the list to complete the sentences below.

catheter   catheterization   colostomy
constipation   defecation   diarrhea
enema   fecal impaction   fecal incontinence
flatulence   flatus   ileostomy
micturition   urinary incontinence   urination
voiding

1. A _____ is an artificial opening between the colon and abdomen.
2. The inability to control the passage of urine is known as _____ _____.
3. _____ is the frequent passage of liquid stools.
4. Gas or air in the stomach or intestines is called _____.
5. A _____ is a tube used to drain or inject fluid through an opening in the body.
6. Three terms that are used to mean the process of emptying the bladder are _____, _____, and _____.
7. _____, the process of inserting a catheter into the urinary bladder, would be performed by a doctor or a nurse.
8. The prolonged retention and accumulation of fecal material in the rectum and lower colon is known as _____ _____.
9. A/an _____ is the introduction of fluid into the rectum and lower colon.
10. _____ — the passage of a hard, dry stool — is common in the elderly and may be quite painful.
11. Bowel movement or _____ is the process of excreting feces through the anus.

ELIMINATION

12. The inability to control the passage of feces and gas through the anus is _____ _____.
13. _____ is the excessive formation of gas in the stomach and intestines.
14. The artificial opening between the ileum and the abdomen is called a/an _____.

TRUE AND FALSE Mark the statement "T" for true or "F" for false. Change the false statements to make them true.

_____ 1. Urine that is light yellow in color should be reported.
_____ 2. A urinal should be left within the client's reach and emptied at the end of the day.
_____ 3. A Foley catheter is the same as an indwelling catheter.
_____ 4. A urine collection bag needs to be kept at the same level as the bladder to allow the urine to drain.
_____ 5. A catheter should be taped to the client's thigh to prevent excessive movement and friction.
_____ 6. Catheter care is the same as perineal care.
_____ 7. Bladder training is used for clients with indwelling catheters only.
_____ 8. Each client should have a bowel movement every day.
_____ 9. A diet high in residue causes constipation.
_____ 10. A colostomy is a permanent opening between the colon and the abdomen.
_____ 11. An ileostomy drains liquid fecal material constantly.

MULTIPLE CHOICE Select the correct word or group of words in parentheses to complete each statement.

1. Adults normally eliminate about (*100 to 150 ml, 1000 to 1500 ml, 2000 to 3000 ml*) of urine a day.
2. Coffee, tea, and alcohol cause the body to produce (*more, less*) urine.
3. When a person perspires heavily, (*more, less*) urine is produced.
4. It should be reported if a client voids less than (*600 ml, 1200 ml, 3000 ml*) in 24 hours.
5. Bedpans, urinals, and commodes need to be cleaned with (*a deodorant, alcohol, a disinfectant*) after each use.
6. The (*smaller, larger*) end of a fracture pan is placed under the buttocks for clients with casts or in traction.
7. If possible, the male client should (*sit, lie down, stand*) when using the urinal.

8. Care of the client with an indwelling catheter is aimed at preventing (*urinary incontinence, bleeding, infection*).
9. Bladder training involves having the client use the toilet, bedpan, or urinal (*at regular intervals, whenever the urge to void is felt, after each meal*).
10. Bleeding in the stomach causes (*dark brown, red, black*) stools to be passed.
11. Stool that is black and sticky is reported as being (*chalky, putty-like, tarry*).
12. Gas-forming foods include (*onions, fruits, meats*).
13. Small amounts of liquid feces pass around the hardened fecal mass and leak from the anus of clients with (*flatulence, diarrhea, fecal impaction*).
14. A colostomy appliance or bag needs to be changed (*whenever it becomes soiled, every 2 to 4 days, every 4 to 6 hours*).
15. Feces from a/an (*ileostomy, colostomy*) contains digestive juices and is very irritating if allowed to contact the skin.

CHECKING UP ON PROCEDURES

Number the following statements to show the order for performing these procedures.

Giving the Client the Bedpan

_____ Clean the genital area if the client cannot do so.
_____ Position the client on the back and have him or her flex the knees and raise the buttocks.
_____ Slide the bedpan out from under the client.
_____ Make sure the client is correctly positioned on the bedpan.
_____ Slide the bedpan under the client.

Catheter Care

_____ Separate the labia (female) or retract the foreskin if the male is uncircumcised.
_____ Make sure the catheter is taped properly.
_____ Perform perineal care.
_____ Apply soap to the cotton balls or gauze pads.
_____ Clean from the meatus down the catheter about 4 inches.

ELIMINATION

Emptying a Urinary Drainage Bag

_____ Place the graduate under the drain of the collection bag.
_____ Open the clamp on the drain.
_____ Put on the gloves.
_____ Allow all urine to drain into the graduate.
_____ Measure the urine.
_____ Close the clamp, and replace the clamped drain in the holder on the bag.

Caring for the Client with a Colostomy

_____ Clean the skin around the stoma with water, rinse, and pat dry, then apply karaya powder or other skin barrier.
_____ Remove the appliance gently.
_____ Apply the appliance so that it is centered over the stoma and use gentle pressure to seal.
_____ Place the waterproof pad under the client's buttocks and disconnect the appliance from the belt.
_____ Peel back the protector from the adhesive surface of the new appliance.
_____ Wipe around the stoma with toilet tissue to remove any mucus or fecal material.

EQUIPMENT LIST

Circle the item in each group that is NOT needed to perform the procedures listed in the heading.

1. **Connecting a leg bag:**
   Alcohol packets
   Cotton balls
   Waterproof protector
   Disposable gloves
   Cap or sterile 4 x 4

2. **Applying a condom catheter:**
   Disposable gloves
   Condom catheter
   Alcohol packets
   Collection bag
   Perineal care equipment

3. **Giving a commercial enema:**
   Waterproof bed protector
   Disposable gloves
   Soap and basin of water
   Toilet tissue
   Bath blanket

4. **Ileostomy care:**
   Cotton balls
   Prescribed solvent
   Bedpan
   Disposable gloves
   Gauze dressing

RECORDING AND REPORTING

Place an "X" on the line before each observation that needs to be reported to your supervisor and recorded.

_____ 1. Client voids before each meal, at bedtime, and upon awakening.
_____ 2. Client's urine has a strong odor of ammonia.
_____ 3. Client has bowel movement every other morning.
_____ 4. Client's stool is light brown.
_____ 5. Client's urine is orange.
_____ 6. Client's stool is hard and streaked with blood.
_____ 7. Client's abdomen is soft.
_____ 8. Client urinates about 30 ml every half hour.
_____ 9. Client is asking to have an enema.
_____ 10. Client needs to get up in the night to urinate.

HIDDEN WORD SEARCH

Write the correct word from the clues given on the broken lines. When you finish, the hidden word will appear by reading vertically.

1. Device used to void in bed
2. Adhesive bag placed over stoma
3. Bowel movement
4. Chair with bedpan
5. Left from food; bulk
6. Fluid into the rectum and colon
7. Type of powder, ring for ostomies
8. Surgical creation of bowel opening
9. Voiding, urination
10. Cone-shaped solid medication
11. Container used by men to void

CHAPTER 16

Collecting Specimens

TERMS TO KNOW Match the terms listed in Column A with the correct definition from Column B.

Column A

_____ 1. Acetone
_____ 2. Calculi
_____ 3. Diabetes mellitus
_____ 4. Glucosuria
_____ 5. Ketone body
_____ 6. Sputum

Column B

a. Sugar in the urine
b. Mucus secreted by the lungs, bronchi, and trachea during respiratory illnesses or disorders
c. Ketone bodies that appear in urine due to rapid breakdown of fat for energy
d. Another term for acetone
e. Stones
f. Chronic disease in which the pancreas fails to secrete enough insulin

TRUE AND FALSE Mark the statement "T" for true or "F" for false. Change the false statements to make them true.

_____ 1. Your client needs to collect three stool specimens. You may use the same container for all the samples.
_____ 2. Urine specimens should not contain toilet tissue.
_____ 3. The routine urine specimen is also called the clean-catch urine sample.
_____ 4. A routine urine specimen must be collected from the first voiding of the morning.

_____ 5. A midstream urine specimen is the same as a clean-voided specimen.

_____ 6. In a clean-catch urine specimen, perineal care is done after the client voids.

_____ 7. In a 24-hour urine specimen, the last voiding of the client is discarded.

_____ 8. A 24-hour urine specimen will have to be restarted if any voiding is spilled or discarded.

_____ 9. You discover a stone while straining a client's urine. The stone and the urine need to be sent to the laboratory.

_____ 10. A fresh-fractional urine specimen is the same as a double-voided specimen.

_____ 11. Stool specimens may contain urine.

_____ 12. Sputum and saliva are different bodily fluids.

MULTIPLE CHOICE Select the correct word or group of words in parentheses to complete each statement.

1. A 24-hour urine specimen needs to be kept (*warm, cool, at room temperature*) during the collection period.

2. During a fresh-fractional urine specimen, the client voids to empty the bladder, then voids again in (*15, 30, 60*) minutes.

3. Diabetes mellitus is a disease in which the (*pancreas, liver, blood*) fails to secrete enough insulin.

4. Urine tests for diabetic clients are usually done (*once, twice, four times*) each day.

5. (*Fresh-fractional, random sample, midstream*) urine specimens are best for testing urine for sugar and ketones.

6. When performing a Clinitest, (*5, 10, 15*) drops of urine are used in the test tube.

7. Keto-Diastix tests for (*blood, sugar and acetone, sugar*) in the urine.

8. The best time to collect a sputum specimen is (*early in the morning, after a meal, before bedtime*).

9. The client should rinse out his or her mouth with (*water, salt solution, mouthwash*) before collecting a sputum specimen.

10. All specimen containers should be (*refrigerated, taken directly to a laboratory, labeled with the client's personal information*).

COLLECTING SPECIMENS

CHECKING UP ON PROCEDURES

Number the following statements to show the order for performing these procedures.

Collecting a Clean-catch Urine Specimen

_____ Ask the client to urinate into the receptacle and then stop the stream.

_____ Ask the client to stop the stream when urine has been collected, then allow him or her to finish.

_____ Hold the specimen container under the client.

_____ Provide perineal care using towelettes or a specified solution.

_____ Ask the client to start urinating again.

_____ Keep the labia separated in the female or the foreskin retracted in the uncircumcised male until the specimen has been collected.

Collecting a Urine Specimen From an Infant

_____ Remove the child's diaper and dispose of it properly.

_____ Remove the adhesive backing from the collection bag and apply to the perineum.

_____ Clean the perineal area.

_____ Diaper the child.

_____ Position the child on the back, knees flexed, and legs separated.

Testing Urine: Testape

_____ Dip about 1/4 inch of the Testape into the specimen and remove it.

_____ Read the number of the color that matches the Testape.

_____ Wait 60 seconds.

_____ Tear about 1 1/2 inches of Testape from the dispenser.

_____ Hold the Testape so that the tested part is downward.

_____ Compare the darkest area of the Testape with the color chart on the dispenser.

Testing Urine: Clinitest

_____ Wait 15 seconds after the boiling has stopped, then shake gently.

_____ Add 10 drops of water to the test tube.

_____ Match the color of the liquid with the color chart.

_____ Place five drips of urine in the test tube.

_____ Drop one tablet into the test tube.

Testing Urine: Keto-Diastix

_____ Remove the stop from the urine after 2 seconds.
_____ Dip the strip into the urine.
_____ Compare the strip with the color chart for glucose after 30 seconds.
_____ Tap the edge of the strip gently against the specimen container.
_____ Wait 15 seconds, then compare the strip with the color chart on the bottle for ketones.

Collecting a Sputum Specimen

_____ Collect one to two tablespoons of sputum.
_____ Ask the client to take two to three deep breaths and cough up the sputum.
_____ Put the lid on the container immediately.
_____ Ask the client to rinse the mouth out with clear water.
_____ Have the client expectorate the sputum directly into the container.
_____ Have the client hold the container if able.

COLLECTING SPECIMENS

CROSSWORD PUZZLE

Complete the crossword puzzle by using the clues below.

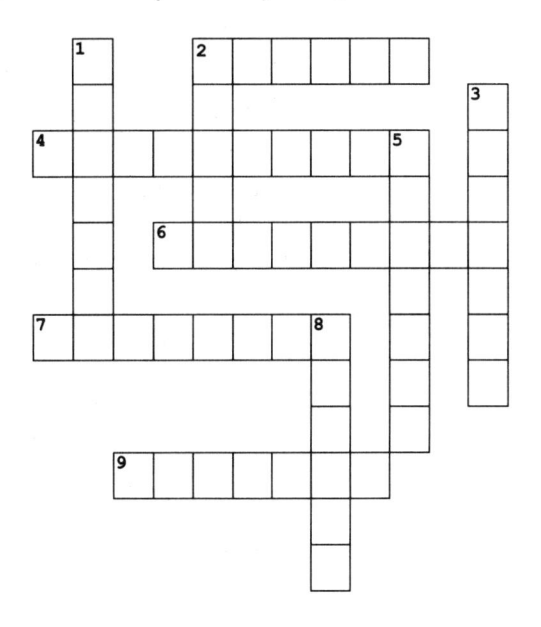

Across:
2. Mucus from the respiratory passages
4. Sugar in the urine
6. Tablet used to test urine for sugar
7. _____ mellitus
9. Secreted by pancreas for sugar breakdown

Down:
1. Stones, as found in the urine
2. Fecal sample
3. Special strip of paper used to test urine for sugar
5. Ketone bodies
8. Clear, thin liquid produced by glands in the mouth

CHAPTER 17

Foods and Fluids

TERMS TO KNOW Using the list below, write the term on the line with the correct definition.

anorexia   calorie   dehydration
dysphagia   edema   intake
nutrient   nutrition   output

_____ 1. The many processes involved in eating, digesting, absorbing, and using foods and fluids
_____ 2. A decrease in the amount of water in body tissues
_____ 3. The amount of fluid taken in by the body
_____ 4. Loss of appetite
_____ 5. Difficulty or discomfort in swallowing
_____ 6. The fluid lost from the body
_____ 7. The amount of energy produced when food is broken down for use
_____ 8. Swelling of body tissues with water
_____ 9. A substance that is ingested, digested, absorbed, and used by the body

TRUE AND FALSE Mark the statement "T" for true or "F" for false. Change the false statements to make them true.

_____ 1. No one food or food group provides all the essential nutrients.
_____ 2. Foods high in fat are usually the most expensive.
_____ 3. Carbohydrate foods include milk, eggs, nuts, and pork.
_____ 4. Vitamins can be ingested through food or produced by the body.
_____ 5. A well-balanced diet includes foods from each of the four food groups.

FOODS AND FLUIDS

      _____ 6. A client with no dietary restrictions is given a general diet.
      _____ 7. Clients on a full liquid diet may not have ice cream.
      _____ 8. Sodium causes the body to retain water.
      _____ 9. Water is the most important physical need for survival.
      _____ 10. Infants and young children need more fluids than adults.
      _____ 11. When the client is NPO, oral hygiene is not allowed.
      _____ 12. Intake and output is recorded in ounces.

MULTIPLE CHOICE   Select the correct word or group of words in parentheses to complete each statement.

1. The most important nutrient, (*fat, carbohydrate, protein*), is necessary for growth and repair of tissue.
2. Each gram of fat provides (*4, 9, 16*) calories.
3. A good source of Vitamin C is (*strawberries, eggs, peas*).
4. Sunlight provides a source of Vitamin (*A, D, K*).
5. A serving of meat is considered to be (*2 to 3, 4 to 6, 10 to 12*) ounces.
6. Appetite usually (*increases, decreases*) during illness and recovery periods.
7. The average daily intake of sodium is (*100 mg, 1000 mg, 3000 mg*) even though the body needs less than half that amount.
8. A diet that is mechanically and chemically nonirritating and low in roughage is the (*soft, bland, low-calorie*) diet.
9. The diabetic diet controls the amount of (*carbohydrate, fiber, salt*) eaten by the client.
10. If storage space is not a problem, (*daily, weekly*) grocery shopping is the most convenient.
11. The ingredient label of a food product lists the (*smallest, largest*) quantity ingredient first.
12. To be a "significant source" of a nutrient, the food must contain at least (*5, 10, 25*) percent of the U. S. recommended daily allowance.
13. Less tender cuts of meat should be cooked using (*dry, moist*) cooking methods.
14. When feeding a client, you should use a (*spoon, fork, special tube*).
15. The client has juice and milk to drink for breakfast. He will need (*1, 2, 3*) straw(s).
16. Vomiting, diarrhea, and bleeding are common causes of (*edema, dehydration*).
17. Client's kept NPO before a scheduled surgery or test are given nothing by mouth beginning at (*8 P.M., midnight, 4 A.M.*) the night before.

LIST

Complete the chart below by supplying the correct information about the Basic Four Food Groups.

Food Group	Examples of Foods	Servings (Adult)	Nutrients
Milk/dairy	_____	_____	_____
	_____		_____
	_____		
_____	Beef, fish	_____	_____
	Poultry		_____
	Peanut butter		
_____	_____	4 or more	_____
	_____		_____
	_____		
_____	_____	_____	Proteins,
	_____		carbohydrates
	_____		B vitamins

CHECKING UP ON PROCEDURES

Number the following statements to show the order for performing this procedure.

Feeding the Client

_____ Converse with the client in a pleasant manner.
_____ Prepare the food for eating.
_____ Drape a napkin across the client's chest and underneath the chin.
_____ Tell the client what kind of foods are on the tray and serve them in the order preferred by the client.
_____ Wipe the client's mouth with a napkin.

MATCHING

Match the nutrient in Column A with the correct function in Column B.

Part 1.   *Column A*   *Column B*

_____ 1. Vitamin C   a. Allows red blood cells to carry oxygen
_____ 2. Vitamin K   b. Tooth and bone formation
_____ 3. Calcium   c. Thyroid gland function; growth
_____ 4. Iron   d. Resistance to infection
_____ 5. Iodine   e. Blood clotting

FOODS AND FLUIDS 77

Part 2. Match the therapeutic diet with the correct description.

Column A	Column B
___ 1. Clear liquid	a. No diet restriction
___ 2. Full liquid	b. Limited amount of fat with increased protein and carbohydrates
___ 3. Soft	c. Fluids that do not leave a residue
___ 4. General	d. Semisolid foods that are easily digested
___ 5. Low-cholesterol	e. Foods that are liquid at room temperature or that melt at body temperature

LIST

Give the correct term for each abbreviation listed.

1. cc _____
2. IV _____
3. NG tube _____
4. TPN _____
5. I & O _____
6. ml _____
7. NPO _____
8. FF _____

HIDDEN WORD SEARCH

Write the correct word from the clues given on the broken lines. When you finish, the hidden word will appear by reading vertically.

1. Diabetic food "groups"   _ _ _ _ _ O _ _ _
2. Meal "list"; what's on the   _ _ _ _ O
3. Nutrient for tissue growth   _ _ _ _ O _ _ _
4. When output exceeds intake   _ _ _ _ _ _ O _ _ _
5. Calcium, sodium, iodine   _ _ O _ _ _ _ _ _
6. Oils, butter, lard are   _ _ O _
7. A, D, E, K, B, C, E are   _ O _ _ _ _ _ _
8. Energy nutrient   _ _ _ _ O _ _ _ _ _ _
9. Fluid taken into body   _ _ O _ _ _ _

CHAPTER 18

Special Procedures

TERMS TO KNOW Supply the correct term from the list to complete the sentences below.

constrict dilate medication
prescription drug over-the-counter drug side effect

1. A drug that can be purchased without a doctor's order is known as a/an _____ _____.
2. When blood vessels _____, they become narrow and blood flow decreases.
3. A chemical substance used to treat disease is called a _____.
4. A drug order that is filled by a pharmacist is called a/an _____ _____.
5. Blood vessels _____ when they expand or open wider and allow greater amounts of blood to flow.
6. Becoming dizzy and faint after taking a medicine for pain is an example of a _____ _____.

TRUE AND FALSE Mark the statement "T" for true or "F" for false. Change the false statements to make them true.

_____ 1. Home health aides do not administer prescription drugs.
_____ 2. Over-the-counter drugs, such as aspirin, may be given to clients by the home health aide.
_____ 3. A suppository melts at room temperature.
_____ 4. Prepoured medications help reduce drug errors by having the dose for a particular time ready for the client to take.
_____ 5. Clients receiving oxygen through a nasal catheter need frequent oral hygiene and nasal care.

SPECIAL PROCEDURES

      6. Home health aides can apply cold but not heat applications.
      7. If the cover of a hot water bottle becomes moist with perspiration, the danger of burns to the client decreases.
      8. Heat lamps are never covered with bed linens or plastic materials.
      9. Heat applications are useful immediately after an injury.
     10. Vital signs are taken before, during, and after a cold sponge bath.

MULTIPLE CHOICE Select the correct word or group of words in parentheses to complete each statement.

1. How a drug will be taken into the body is known as the (*form, dose, route*).
2. Drugs applied directly to the skin are called (*subcutaneous, topical, oral*) medications.
3. (*Oral, Sublingual, Topical*) drugs are placed under the tongue to be absorbed.
4. A (*capsule, tablet, lozenge*) is a small container that holds a powder or liquid medication.
5. Death occurs within (*2, 4, 8*) minutes if breathing stops.
6. The most common device used in giving oxygen is the (*nasal catheter, nasal cannula, face mask*).
7. (*Heat, Cold*) causes blood vessels to expand.
8. The effects of heat are greater and occur faster with (*dry, moist*) heat applications.
9. Moist heat applications are applied for (*5, 20, 60*) minutes.
10. Immersing the pelvic area in warm water is called a (*hot soak, Sitz bath, sponge bath*).
11. In dry heat applications, (*higher, lower*) temperatures are used than in moist heat applications.
12. An example of a dry heat application is (*hot compress, hot soak, hot water bottle*).
13. An ice bag is a (*moist, dry*) cold application.
14. A cold compress needs to be changed when it becomes warm, usually every (*5, 10, 20*) minutes.
15. A cold sponge bath should last (*10, 25, 45*) minutes.

CHECKING UP ON PROCEDURES

Number the statements to show the order for performing these procedures.

Assisting with Medications

_____ Loosen container lids, tops, or caps and tell the client the names of each medication.
_____ Help the client wash his or her hands.
_____ Check the prescription label.
_____ Assist the client with the medication(s).
_____ Place the medication(s) within the client's reach.

Applying an Ice Bag

_____ Fill the bag one-half to two-thirds full with crushed ice.
_____ Place the bag in the flannel cover or towel.
_____ Place the cap or stopper on securely.
_____ Fill the bag with water, close, check for leaks, and empty.
_____ Apply the bag to the area.

EQUIPMENT LIST

Circle the item in each group that is NOT needed to perform the procedure listed in the heading.

1. **Applying a cold compress:**
   Large basin with ice
   Large basin with cold water
   Small basin with cold water
   Washcloths
   Waterproof pad

2. **Giving a cold sponge bath:**
   Bath basin
   Bath thermometer
   Bath towels and washcloths
   Large basin with ice
   Thermometer

3. **Applying an ice bag:**
   Ice collar (or bag)
   Flannel cover or towel
   Crushed or chipped ice
   Paper towels
   Bath thermometer

SPECIAL PROCEDURES

LIST

1. List the "five rights" for safely taking medications:

   a. _____
   b. _____
   c. _____
   d. _____
   e. _____

2. Name four reasons for stopping a cold sponge bath and notifying the nurse:

   a. _____
   b. _____
   c. _____
   d. _____

3. List the meaning for each abbreviation below:

   a. q.d.   _____
   b. q.6h. _____
   c. q.i.d. _____
   d. p.c.   _____
   e. b.i.d. _____
   f. p.r.n. _____
   g. q.o.d. _____

4. List three danger signals that must be reported immediately if seen in clients receiving heat applications.

   a. _____
   b. _____
   c. _____

5. List five signs or symptoms of complications from cold application that should be reported immediately.

   a. _____
   b. _____
   c. _____
   d. _____
   e. _____

CHAPTER 19

The Postoperative Client

TERMS TO KNOW Match the term listed in Column A with the correct definition in Column B.

Column A

____ 1. Atelectasis
____ 2. Binder
____ 3. Dressing
____ 4. Elastic bandage
____ 5. Elastic stockings
____ 6. Embolus
____ 7. Postoperative
____ 8. Preoperative
____ 9. Thrombus
____ 10. Wound

Column B

a. A blood clot
b. A blood clot that travels
c. Damage to skin and underlying tissues
d. Collapse of a portion of the lung
e. After surgery
f. Gauze bandage that covers a wound
g. Used to promote comfort, give support, and hold dressings in place
h. Before surgery
i. TED hose
j. Provide support and reduce swelling to extremities after injury

TRUE AND FALSE Mark the statement "T" for true or "F" for false. Change the false statements to make them true.

____ 1. Fears are common in clients before and after surgery.
____ 2. You should answer any question the client asks about his or her surgery and diagnosis.
____ 3. The care of the postoperative client centers on promoting comfort and preventing complications.

THE POSTOPERATIVE CLIENT

_____ 4. All clients will have pain after surgery.
_____ 5. A decubitus ulcer is an example of a wound.
_____ 6. Not all wounds need to be covered with a dressing.
_____ 7. The home health aide is responsible for changing dressings.
_____ 8. Some postoperative clients need to be repositioned every two hours.
_____ 9. Coughing and deep-breathing exercises are not painful for the client.
_____ 10. TED hose, or elastic stockings, are applied before the client gets out of bed.
_____ 11. Elastic bandages are applied from the top of the limb to the lower part of the limb.
_____ 12. If possible, fingers or toes should not be exposed when applying elastic bandages.

MULTIPLE CHOICE Select the correct word or group of words in parentheses to complete each statement.

1. The surgical wound is called a/an (*suture, decubitus, incision*).
2. Supplies for dressings must be kept (*clean, sterile*).
3. The preferred position of the client for coughing and deep-breathing exercises is usually the (*semi-Fowler's, supine, prone*) position.
4. When coughing, the client is encouraged to keep the mouth (*closed, open*), while supporting the incision.
5. The client doing deep-breathing exercises should take a total of (*2, 5, 10*) deep breaths.
6. Leg exercises are done by the client in the (*standing, supine, semi-Fowler's*) position.
7. Straight abdominal binders are used for (*abdominal support, preventing blood clots*).
8. A rectangular binder with tails attached to each side is a (*breast, T, scultetus*) binder.
9. When applying a binder, fasten pins so that they point (*toward, away from*) the incision.
10. Elastic stockings need to be removed at least (*1, 2, 4*) time(s) a day.
11. If a client complains of pain and tingling in the leg when elastic stockings are worn, you should (*remove the stockings, exercise the leg, call the doctor*).
12. When wrapping elastic bandages, each turn should overlap about (*one-third, one-half, two-thirds*) of the previous turn.

CHECKING UP ON PROCEDURES

Number the statements to show the order for performing these procedures.

Coughing and Deep-breathing Exercises

Have the client deep breathe:

_____ Ask the client to take a breath as deep as possible.
_____ Ask the client to hold the breath for three to five seconds.
_____ Have the client place his or her hands over the rib cage.
_____ Ask the client to exhale slowly through pursed lips until the ribs move as far down as possible.
_____ Ask the client to exhale until the ribs move as far down as possible.

Applying Elastic Stockings

_____ Make sure the stocking is not twisted and has no creases or wrinkles.
_____ Support the client's foot at the heel.
_____ Hold the foot and heel of the stocking and gather up the rest of the stocking in your hands.
_____ Slip the foot of the stocking over the client's toes, foot, and heel.
_____ Pull the stocking up over the leg.

Applying Elastic Bandages

_____ Apply the bandage to the smallest part of the extremity.
_____ Apply the bandage smoothly with firm, even pressure.
_____ Pin, tape, or clip the end of the bandage to hold it in place.
_____ Make overlapping spiral turns in an upward direction.
_____ Make two circular turns around the part.

LABELING

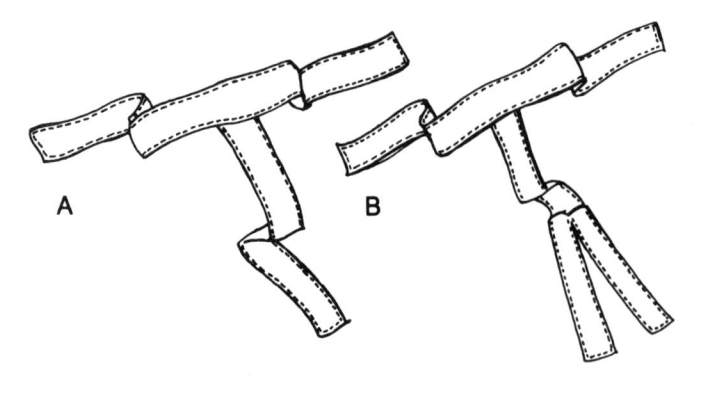

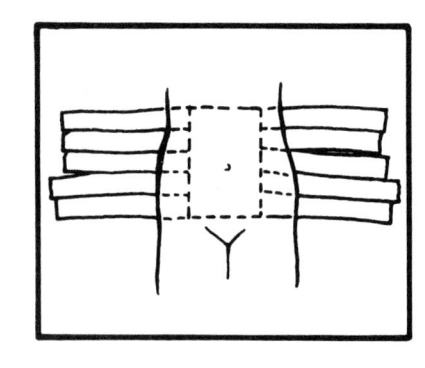

Identify the binders below.

Fig. 19–1. _____   Fig. 19–2. _____

THE POSTOPERATIVE CLIENT
85

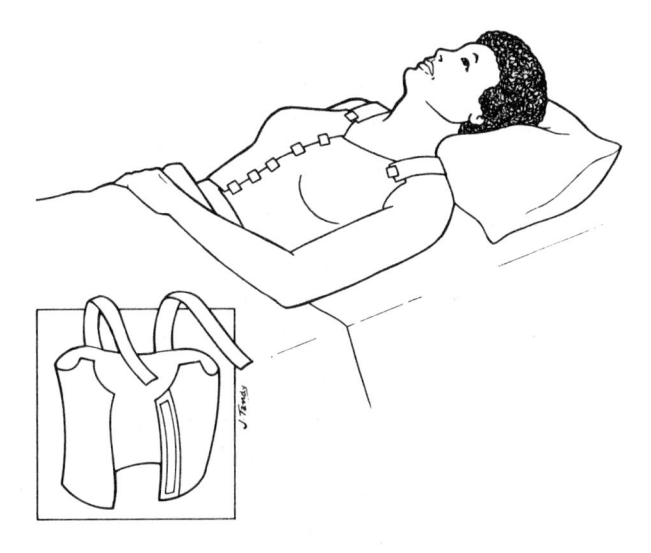

Fig. 19–3. _____

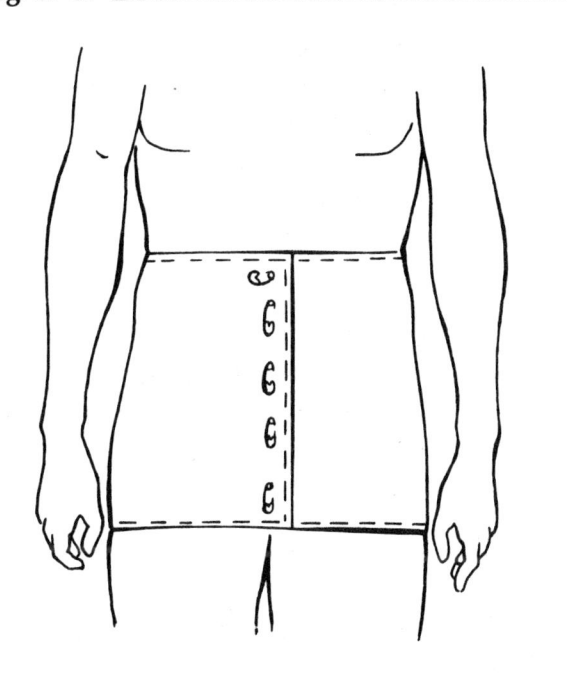

Fig. 19–4. _____

CHAPTER 20

The Mother and Her Newborn

TERMS TO KNOW Using the list below, write the term on the line with the correct definition.

bubbling   circumcision   rooting reflex
sterilization   umbilical cord

_____ 1. The process of destroying all microorganisms
_____ 2. Burping or releasing air from the stomach
_____ 3. The baby turns his or her head in the direction of a stimulus
_____ 4. Surgical removal of the foreskin
_____ 5. The structure that carries blood, oxygen, and nutrients from the mother to the fetus.

TRUE AND FALSE Mark the statement "T" for true or "F" for false. Change the false statements to make them true.

_____ 1. Responding quickly to an infant's cry helps the child feel safe and secure.
_____ 2. Cribs for infants should not have pillows.
_____ 3. Mothers need to wash their nipples with soap and water before each breast-feeding.
_____ 4. Mothers who breast-feed should be encouraged to nurse from one breast at a feeding.
_____ 5. Milk is added to powdered and concentrated formula.
_____ 6. Burp an infant about halfway through the bottle feeding.

_____ 7. Breast-fed infants do not need to burp.
_____ 8. The umbilical cord stump needs to be kept dry.
_____ 9. When the cord falls off, the infant may have a sponge bath.
_____ 10. After circumcision, the penis of an infant will look red and swollen.
_____ 11. The circumcision area is cleaned at each diaper change with alcohol.
_____ 12. Start an infant's bath by washing the eyes first.

MULTIPLE CHOICE Select the correct word or group of words in parentheses to complete each statement.

1. Neck support is necessary for infants for the first (*month, 3 months, year*) of life.
2. Breast-fed infants may need to nurse every (*2 to 3, 3 to 4, 4 to 6*) hours.
3. The diet of the breast-feeding mother needs to include foods high in (*fiber, carbohydrates, calcium*).
4. Formula prepared ahead may be safely stored in the refrigerator for up to (*12, 24, 36*) hours.
5. When sterilizing baby bottles, boil the pot for (*5, 15, 30*) minutes.
6. Formula remaining in a bottle after a feeding should be (*saved for the next feeding, discarded*).
7. Cloth diapers are folded so that the extra thickness is placed in the (*front, back*) for baby girls.
8. The diaper needs to be (*above, below*) the umbilical cord stump.
9. Pins on cloth diapers should point (*toward, away from*) the abdomen of the infant.
10. The cord stump will dry and fall off in (*3 to 5, 7 to 10, 10 to 14*) days from birth.
11. Bath water temperature for a baby's bath should not exceed (*90, 100, 105*) degrees Fahrenheit.
12. Hold the infant in the (*cradle, shoulder, football*) hold to shampoo the head.

88 MOSBY'S WORKBOOK FOR THE HOMEMAKER/HOME HEALTH AIDE

CHECKING UP ON PROCEDURES

Number the statements to show the correct order for performing these procedures.

Sterilizing Bottles

_____ Pour about two inches of water into the sterilizer or pot.
_____ Rinse all equipment thoroughly in hot water.
_____ Wash equipment in hot soapy water.
_____ Put all equipment into the sterilizer or pot.
_____ Bring the water to a boil.

Diapering a Baby

_____ Unfasten the dirty diaper.
_____ Raise the baby's legs and slide a clean diaper under the buttocks.
_____ Give cord care, and clean the circumcision.
_____ Secure the diaper in place.
_____ Clean the genital area from front to back, rinse, and pat dry.
_____ Bring the back of the diaper over the front.

LABELING

Name the infant holds shown in Figures 1–3 below.

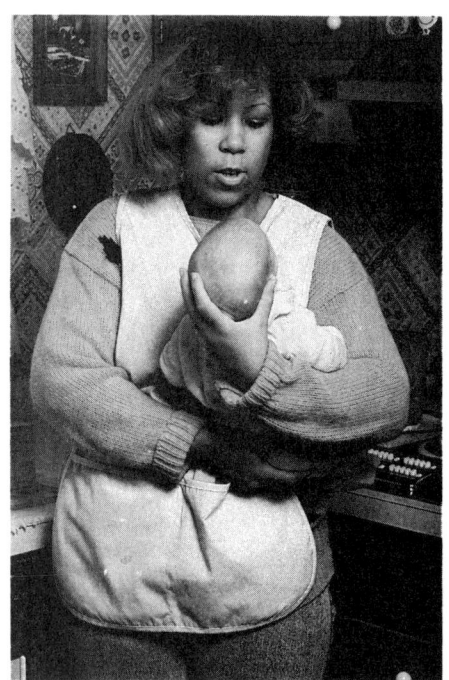

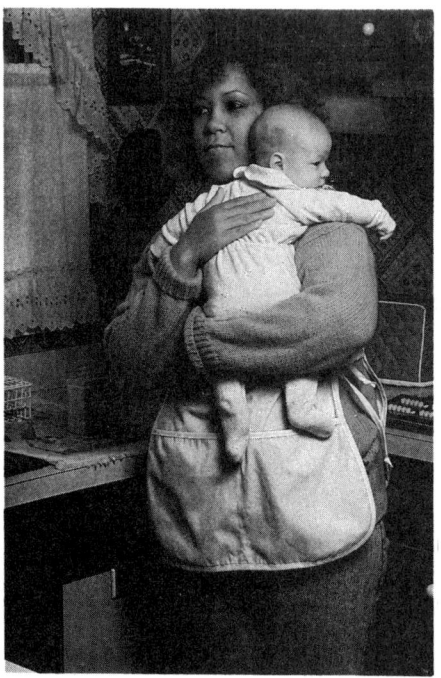

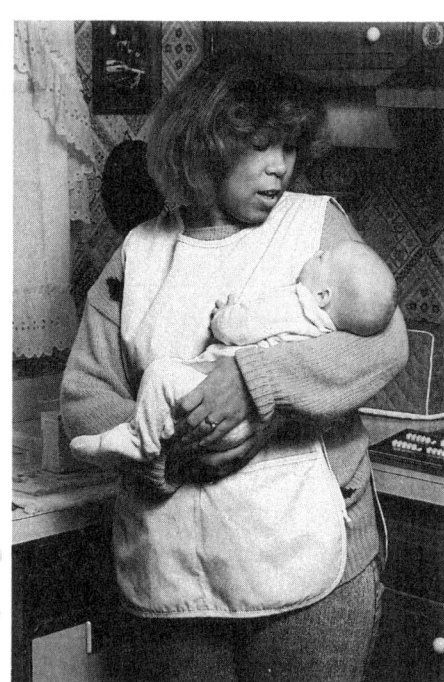

FIG. 20–1. _____   FIG. 20–2. _____   FIG. 20–3. _____

LIST

List 10 signs or symptoms of illness in an infant that should be reported:

1. _____
2. _____
3. _____
4. _____
5. _____
6. _____
7. _____
8. _____
9. _____
10. _____

CHAPTER 21

Common Health Problems

TERMS TO KNOW   Supply the correct term from the list to complete the sentences below.

amputation
compound fracture
malignant tumor
tumor
benign tumor
fracture
metastasis
closed fracture
gangrene
stroke

1. _____ occurs when tissue dies and becomes black, cold, and shriveled.
2. A new growth of abnormal cells, either benign or malignant is called a _____.
3. A _____ _____ grows slowly and within a localized area and usually does not cause death.
4. A tumor that grows rapidly and invades other tissues — one that may cause death if not treated — is a _____ _____.
5. Often caused by falls and accidents, a _____ is a broken bone.
6. _____ is the removal of all or part of an extremity.
7. A simple fracture, also called a/an _____, occurs when the bone is broken but the skin is intact.
8. When a bone is broken and comes through the skin, it is called an open or _____ _____.
9. _____ is the spread of cancer to other parts of the body.
10. When the blood supply to a part of the brain is suddenly interrupted, the client is said to have suffered a/an _____.

COMMON HEALTH PROBLEMS

TRUE AND FALSE Mark the statement "T" for true or "F" for false. Change the false statements to make them true.

1. Clients with cancer may be treated by surgery, radiation, drugs, or a combination of these methods.
2. Chemotherapy can produce harsh side effects.
3. Closed reduction of a bone fracture involves surgery.
4. A dry cast is gray and cool and has a musty smell.
5. Continuous traction can be removed at times ordered by the doctor.
6. Clients in traction are usually allowed only the back-lying position.
7. Following a hip pinning, the client will need to keep the operated leg adducted while lying in bed.
8. Clients with osteoporosis will be placed on bedrest.
9. Clients with Parkinson's disease will have difficulty with movement and self-care activities.
10. Keeping the environment consistent and safe are important for the client with Alzheimer's disease.
11. Be sure to face the hearing impaired client directly when speaking.
12. The client with emphysema usually prefers a semi-Fowler's position for easier breathing.
13. Chest pain that is not relieved by rest or nitroglycerin may be due to a heart attack.
14. Congestive heart failure can lead to pulmonary edema — fluid in the lungs.
15. Insulin shock occurs if a client does not have enough insulin.

MULTIPLE CHOICE Select the word or group of words in parentheses to complete each statement.

1. Clients receiving radiation therapy who develop radiation sickness may need special (*exercises, skin care, oral hygiene*) as ordered by the doctor.
2. Stomatitis is an inflammation of the (*mouth, stomach, bowel*) often resulting from chemotherapy.
3. (*Osteoarthritis, rheumatoid arthritis*) occurs with aging and often affects the hips and knees.
4. Plaster of Paris casts need (*12 to 24, 24 to 48, 36 to 72*) hours to dry.
5. Casts (*should, should not*) be covered with blankets, plastic, or other material during the drying period.

6. When turning or positioning a client with a new cast, use the (*palms of your hands, fingers*) to support the cast and limb.
7. Traction applied directly to a bone is called (*skin, skeletal, intermittent*) traction.
8. Change the bottom linens of the client in traction from (*side to side, bottom to top, top to bottom*).
9. When a client with a hip pinning is allowed to sit in a chair, place a straight-backed chair on the (*unoperated, operated*) side of the bed.
10. A major cause of osteoporosis is a lack of (*iron, calcium, protein*) in the diet.
11. In a spinal cord injury, the (*lower, higher*) the level of injury, the greater the loss of function.
12. With a hearing aid, background noises are (*amplified, eliminated*).
13. The earpiece of a hearing aid should (*be washed daily, never be washed, be cleaned professionally*).
14. A blind person can be recognized by a (*red, white, black*) cane and a guide dog.
15. Clients complaining of sudden, severe chest pain, which is not relieved by rest and nitroglycerin, may be suffering (*congestive heart failure, a stroke, a heart attack*).
16. A diabetic client becomes weak, hungry, dizzy, and confused. He is probably developing (*insulin shock, diabetic coma*).

MATCHING

Match the disease in Column A with the correct description in Column B.

	Column A		*Column B*
_____	1. Alzheimer's disease	a.	Causes air to be trapped in lung, with "barrel chest"
_____	2. Angina pectoris	b.	Increased eye pressure
_____	3. Bronchiectasis	c.	Brain degeneration causing loss of muscle function
_____	4. Congestive heart failure	d.	Elevated blood pressure
_____	5. Emphysema	e.	"Chest pain" relieved by rest and nitroglycerin
_____	6. Glaucoma	f.	Inflammation of lung tissue
_____	7. Hypertension	g.	Bronchi enlarge and collect pus
_____	8. Myocardial infarction	h.	Heart fails to pump
_____	9. Parkinson's disease	i.	Progressive change in brain tissue causing memory loss, poor judgment, moodiness
_____	10. Pneumonia	j.	Heart attack

COMMON HEALTH PROBLEMS

LIST

1. List the seven early warning signs of cancer.

   a. _____
   b. _____
   c. _____
   d. _____
   e. _____
   f. _____
   g. _____

2. Name five signs or symptoms to report immediately when caring for a client in a new cast.

   a. _____
   b. _____
   c. _____
   d. _____
   e. _____

3. Reality orientation is important for clients with chronic brain syndrome. List suggestions to follow regarding:

   a. Greeting the client: _____

   b. Time and place: _____

   c. Daily routines: _____

   d. Instructions: _____

4. List four signs and symptoms of diabetes mellitus.

   a. _____
   b. _____
   c. _____
   d. _____

CROSSWORD PUZZLE

Complete the crossword puzzle using the clues below.

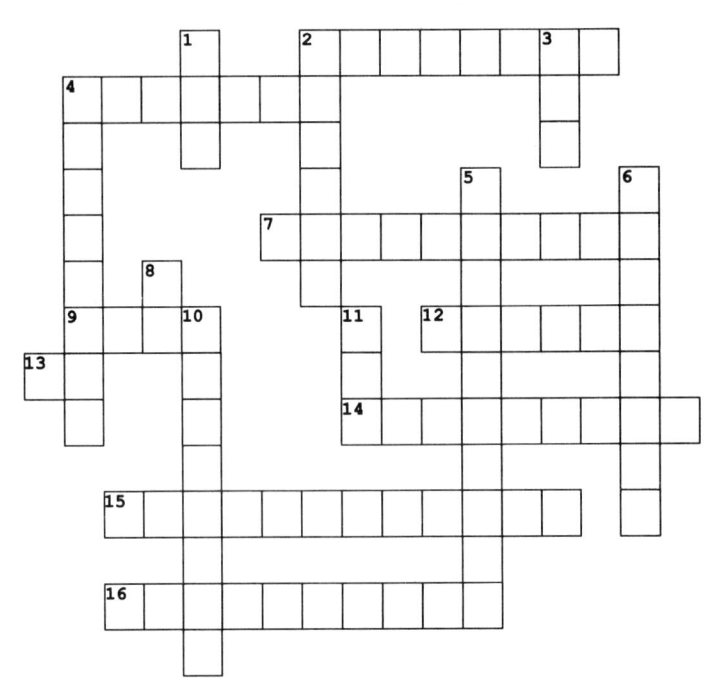

Across:
2. Eye disorder in which the lens becomes cloudy
4. Loss of the ability to speak
7. Excessive bleeding
9. Plaster of Paris, plastic, or fiberglass cover for a broken limb
12. Narrowing of breathing passages causing dyspnea, shortness of breath, wheezing, coughing
13. Myocardial infarction (abbreviation)
14. Inflammation of a joint
15. Disorder causing bones to become porous and brittle
16. Inflammation of the bronchi

Down:
1. Coronary artery disease (abbreviation)
2. A new growth of abnormal cells; malignancy
3. Congestive heart failure (abbreviation)
4. Loss of hair
5. Artificial body part, such as an artificial leg
6. Covering the edge of a cast with tape
8. Multiple sclerosis (abbreviation)
10. Used to immobilize a fracture, pulls in two directions to keep the bone in place
11. Cerebral vascular accident (abbreviation)

CHAPTER 22

Basic Emergency Care

TERMS TO KNOW Match the terms listed in Column A with the correct definition from Column B.

Column A

_____ 1. Cardiac arrest
_____ 2. Convulsion
_____ 3. First aid
_____ 4. Grand mal seizure
_____ 5. Hemorrhage
_____ 6. Petit mal seizure
_____ 7. Poison
_____ 8. Respiratory arrest
_____ 9. Seizure
_____ 10. Shock

Column B

a. A short seizure with loss of consciousness, twitching of arm, face
b. Condition resulting from inadequate blood supply
c. Excessive blood loss
d. Sudden stoppage of breathing and heart action
e. Substance that can harm tissues and cause death
f. Emergency care given before medical help arrives
g. A convulsion
h. Contraction of all muscles at once, followed by jerking movements
i. Violent, sudden tremor or contractions; seizure
j. Stoppage of breathing while heart continues to pump

TRUE AND FALSE

Mark the statement "T" for true or "F" for false. Change the false statements to make them true.

_____ 1. In an emergency, move the victim to a more comfortable location if possible.
_____ 2. Do not give food or fluids to victims of an emergency.
_____ 3. Cardiac arrest can occur without respiratory arrest.
_____ 4. In CPR, blood is circulated by cardiac massage — that is, by compressing the heart between the breastbone and the spinal cord.
_____ 5. The radial pulse is used to check for pulselessness in cardiac arrest.
_____ 6. The Heimlich maneuver is not effective if the victim is unconscious.
_____ 7. Obese victims of airway obstruction will require chest thrusts in place of abdominal thrusts when performing the Heimlich maneuver.
_____ 8. A steady flow of blood usually means bleeding is from an artery.
_____ 9. During a seizure, the client should be lowered to the floor and kept supine.
_____ 10. Burns on the body should be submersed in ice immediately.

MULTIPLE CHOICE

Select the correct word or group of words in parentheses to complete each statement.

1. Victims in an emergency should be kept (*warm, cool*) until help arrives.
2. No pulse, no breathing, and unconsciousness are the major signs of (*seizures, respiratory arrest, cardiac arrest*).
3. In applying the head-tilt/chin-lift maneuver to a child, the neck (*is, is not*) hyperextended.
4. For CPR to be successful, the victim must be placed on a hard surface in the (*prone, supine, side-lying*) position.
5. The heel of the hand is placed on the (*upper, middle, lower*) portion of the sternum [breastbone] for chest compression.
6. For good chest compression, the rescuer's elbows must be (*straight, bent*) and the shoulders must be directly over the victim's chest.
7. Firm downward pressure is applied to depress the sternum (*1/2 to 1, 1 1/2 to 2, 2 to 3 1/2*) inches.

BASIC EMERGENCY CARE

8. Compressions must be given at a rate of (*60 to 70, 80 to 100, 100 plus*) per minute for an adult.
9. CPR begins with (*1, 2, 5*) ventilations.
10. With two rescuers performing CPR, ventilations are given after (*each, 5, 15*) compression(*s*).
11. In infant CPR, compressions are performed with (*the heel of one hand, two to three fingers, the heel of both hands interlaced*).
12. The victim of airway obstruction will (*appear flushed, clutch at the throat, cough excessively*) and be very frightened.
13. In performing the Heimlich maneuver, the abdominal thrusts are directed (*upward, downward, inward*) quickly.
14. The first step in controlling external bleeding is to apply (*direct pressure over, pressure over the artery above*) the bleeding site.
15. (*Petit mal, grand mal*) seizures are the more common.
16. Petit mal seizures usually last (*10 to 20 seconds, 30 to 60 seconds, 1 to 3 minutes*).
17. The client suffering a seizure (*should, should not*) be restrained.
18. Burned areas of the body need to be covered with a (*blanket, wet dressing or sheet, salve or cream for burns*).
19. Do not allow the person who has fainted to get up for about (*3, 5, 15*) minutes after symptoms have disappeared.
20. The stroke victim should be turned onto the (*affected, unaffected*) side.

CHECKING UP ON PROCEDURES

Number the statements to show the order for performing these procedures.

Adult CPR: One Person

_____ Check for breathlessness; give two ventilations.
_____ Logroll the victim to the supine position.
_____ Call for help.
_____ Open the airway using the head-tilt/chin-lift maneuver.
_____ Check for unresponsiveness.
_____ Check for pulselessness; start cardiac compressions.

Clearing the Obstructed Airway: Unconscious Adult

_____ Logroll the victim to the supine position.
_____ Check for unresponsiveness.
_____ Call for help.
_____ Check for breathlessness; give one ventilation.
_____ Do the Heimlich maneuver if unable to ventilate the victim.
_____ Open the airway using the head-tilt/chin-lift maneuver.

Obstructed Airway: Finger Sweep Maneuver

_____ Form a hook with your index finger.
_____ Open the victim's mouth using the tongue-jaw lift maneuver.
_____ Try to dislodge and remove the foreign object, being careful not to push the object deeper into the throat.
_____ Grasp the foreign object if it is within reach.
_____ Insert your index finger into the victim's mouth along the side of the cheek and deep into the throat.

LIST

1. Imagine you are calling to activate the EMS system. Name five important pieces of information that you should be prepared to give:

    a. _____
    b. _____
    c. _____
    d. _____
    e. _____

2. List the "ABCs" of CPR:

    a. A _____
    b. B _____
    c. C _____

3. What are the three steps for establishing breathlessness:

    a. _____
    b. _____
    c. _____

4. Name seven signs of shock:

    a. _____   e. _____
    b. _____   f. _____
    c. _____   g. _____
    d. _____

BASIC EMERGENCY CARE

HIDDEN WORD SEARCH Write the correct word from the clues given on the broken lines. When you finish, the hidden word will appear by reading vertically.

1. Maneuver to relieve choking _ Ⓞ _ _ _ _ _
2. The material vomited _ _ Ⓞ _ _ _ _
3. Paralysis on one side _ _ _ _ _ _ Ⓞ _ _
4. Emergency personnel not EMTs _ _ Ⓞ _ _ _ _ _ _ _
5. To turn the body as a unit _ _ Ⓞ _ _ _
6. Emergency Medical Services Ⓞ _ _
7. Airway obstruction _ _ _ _ _ Ⓞ _
8. Intentional overdose may be _ _ _ Ⓞ _ _ _
9. Bluish color of skin _ Ⓞ _ _ _ _ _ _

CHAPTER 23

The Dying Client

TERMS TO KNOW   Using the list below, match the terms with the correct definition.

autopsy
postmortem
terminal illness
coroner
reincarnation
living will
rigor mortis

_____ 1. The belief that the spirit or soul is reborn in another human body or in another form of life

_____ 2. An illness or injury from which recovery is not expected

_____ 3. Examination of the body after death

_____ 4. After death

_____ 5. A statement expressing a person's desire not to have life prolonged by artificial means

_____ 6. A public official responsible for investigating the cause of death

_____ 7. Stiffness or rigidity of skeletal muscles that occurs after death

TRUE AND FALSE   Mark the statement "T" for true or "F" for false. Change the false statements to make them true.

_____ 1. Hope and the will to live are two very strong psychological forces that influence living and dying.

_____ 2. Living wills are considered legal documents throughout the United States.

_____ 3. If your client has a DNR order, you must activate the EMS system and give basic life support when signs of death are present.

_____ 4. Adults are more fearful about death than children.

_____ 5. All dying clients go through each of the five stages of dying.

_____ 6. Vision is one of the last functions to be lost as death approaches.
_____ 7. You should allow family members to give care to the dying client if they wish to do so.
_____ 8. The coroner may order that an autopsy be performed.
_____ 9. It is not unusual for a dying client to be incontinent of urine or feces.
_____ 10. Showing your feelings to the family of the dead client may be very appropriate.

MULTIPLE CHOICE Select the correct word or group of words in parentheses to complete each statement.

1. Children under the age of (*3, 5, 10*) have no concept of death.
2. Clients in the (*denial, anger, depression*) stage of dying frequently blame others and resent those who are alive and healthy.
3. (*Bargaining, denial, acceptance*) is the stage in which the dying person says, "Yes, me, but . . . ."
4. While in the (*denial, anger, bargaining*) stage, the dying client is not able to deal with problems or decisions about the illness or injury.
5. As the dying client becomes weaker, (*more, less*) care will be needed.
6. As death approaches, body temperature (*falls, rises*).
7. Clients with breathing problems are usually more comfortable in (*side-lying, supine, semi-Fowler's*) position.
8. Blood pressure (*rises, falls*) as death nears.
9. If you are with a client when death occurs, you need to call (*your supervisor, the coroner, the funeral director*).
10. After death, the body needs to be placed in a natural position (*before, after*) rigor mortis sets in.
11. Rigor mortis occurs within (*2 to 4 hours, 12 hours, 1 to 2 days*) after death.
12. Postmortem care is (*always, sometimes, never*) done before the body has been declared dead.

CHECKING UP ON PROCEDURES

Number the following statements to show the order for performing this procedure.

Postmortem Care

_____ Brush and comb the hair if necessary.
_____ Close the eyes and mouth.
_____ Bathe soiled body areas with plain water, dry thoroughly and replace soiled dressings.
_____ Position the body in the supine position with the arms and legs straight.
_____ Put a clean gown on the body.
_____ Remove all jewelry except for wedding rings, which should be secured in place with tape.

LIST

1. List the five stages of dying as identified by Dr. Elisabeth Kubler-Ross:

   a. _____ d. _____
   b. _____ e. _____
   c. _____

2. List the five signs of approaching death:

   a. _____
   b. _____
   c. _____
   d. _____
   e. _____

3. Name four physical signs that death has occurred:

   a. _____
   b. _____
   c. _____
   d. _____

Final Examination

Each question below has one correct answer. Read carefully and select the best choice.

1. Which person would NOT be a good candidate to receive home care services?
   a. An 85-year-old man recovering from hip surgery
   b. A 48-year-old female with terminal cancer
   c. A 31-year-old disabled veteran with partial paralysis
   d. A 66-year-old female with a bowel obstruction
2. In order for a client to receive home care services:
   a. The care must be medically necessary
   b. The client must be terminally ill
   c. The family must be able to pay for the services
   d. The client needs to have been recently hospitalized
3. The number of times you will visit a client is determined by the:
   a. Client's age
   b. Plan of treatment
   c. Client's ability to pay for services
   d. Request of the client or the family
4. In general, the member of the home care team who spends the most time with the client is the:
   a. Registered nurse
   b. Physical therapist
   c. Home health aide
   d. Licensed practical nurse

5. You are assigned to Mrs. S. who needs to have her colostomy bag changed. You have never done this procedure, but Mrs. S. says she can "talk you through it." You should:
   a. Go ahead and change the bag with the client's help
   b. Tell Mrs. S. to change the bag herself
   c. Call your supervisor and ask for help
   d. Review the procedure in your book, then do it

6. Which of the following is NOT permitted of the home health aide while working?
   a. Wearing low heeled, nonskid shoes
   b. Smoking
   c. Taking a prescription drug for a thyroid disorder
   d. Wearing hair that is swept back and off the collar

7. Which of the following is an example of confidential (privileged) information?
   a. Your client is a former Olympic athlete.
   b. Your client is an immigrant from Sweden.
   c. Most of your clients are elderly.
   d. The client you visit on Wednesdays has cancer.

8. A client refuses to stay in bed. The home health aide tells the client if he continues to get up she will have to tie him in bed. This is an example of:
   a. Assault
   b. Battery
   c. False imprisonment
   d. Negligence

9. A home health aide arrives late to a client's home but tells the supervisor she was on time. This is an example of:
   a. Assault
   b. An incident
   c. Unethical behavior
   d. A crime

10. When an incident occurs in the home, you must do all of the following EXCEPT:
    a. Report the incident immediately to your supervisor
    b. Complete an incident report
    c. Check the mental and physical condition of the client
    d. Write a notation in the client's chart that an incident report has been filed

11. An example of feedback is:
    a. Having a client repeat something that you said
    b. A facial expression
    c. Speaking clearly and distinctly to a client
    d. Giving opinions or advice
12. Which is an example of a barrier to communication?
    a. You encourage a client who cannot speak to use paper and pencil to communicate.
    b. Your client begins to talk about dying. You hold his hand and listen to what he says.
    c. You bring along a sports magazine for your client who once coached high school basketball.
    d. Your client is asking a number of questions while you need to leave. You glance at the clock and begin to put on your coat.
13. The prefix "dys" in a medical word means:
    a. Bad, difficult, or abnormal
    b. Separation, away from
    c. Slow
    d. Without or not
14. A medical condition with the ending "itis" means:
    a. Profuse flow or discharge
    b. Enlargement of
    c. Inflammation
    d. Dilation, stretching
15. Your client is to walk a short distance t.i.d. and HS. This means your client will walk:
    a. Twice a day
    b. Before each meal
    c. Every morning and night
    d. Three times a day and at bedtime
16. Phone conversations, visits, observations, treatments and care provided, and the client's response to care are all recorded on the:
    a. Nursing or progress notes
    b. Care plan
    c. Client information sheet
    d. Work plan
17. An example of a sign is:
    a. Pain in the elbow
    b. Bleeding from a wound
    c. Headache
    d. Abdominal cramping

18. An example of a symptom is:
    a. Fatigue
    b. Cough
    c. Diarrhea
    d. Sweating
19. Which observation needs to be reported immediately?
    a. Client's vital signs are in normal limits.
    b. Client has a soft brown stool every other day.
    c. Client has not urinated in 8 hours.
    d. Client is having a regular menstrual period.
20. Your client complains of pain in her right elbow. You notice that the elbow is quite swollen and red. An example of objective recording in this case would be:
    a. Client states, "My right elbow is very painful."
    b. Client's right elbow is painful.
    c. Client has pain and swelling in right elbow.
    d. Client's right elbow is swollen and red.
21. The eustachian tube connects the:
    a. Ovary with the uterus
    b. Middle ear with the throat
    c. Pancreas with the small intestine
    d. Kidney with the bladder
22. The auditory nerve is responsible for:
    a. Hearing
    b. Vision
    c. Taste
    d. Smell
23. Blood returns to the heart through:
    a. Arteries
    b. Veins
    c. Capillaries
    d. The ventricles
24. Urine leaves the body through the:
    a. Bladder
    b. Kidneys
    c. Ureters
    d. Urethra
25. Ovulation normally occurs:
    a. Around day 14 of the menstrual cycle
    b. Around day 28 of the menstrual cycle
    c. Between the ages of 10 and 14 years
    d. As the menstrual cycle begins

26. The most ideal situation for the growth of microorganisms would be in a container of leftover food:
    a. Sealed and frozen
    b. Refrigerated
    c. Sitting on the countertop
    d. Placed in a cooler on a sunny, 88° F day
27. When handwashing with a bar of soap, hold the bar:
    a. Until there is sufficient lather
    b. During the entire procedure
    c. For the first minute
    d. Until you rinse your hands
28. Your client is in isolation. It is important to:
    a. Flush urine and feces immediately down the toilet
    b. Use disposable dishes, cups, and eating utensils for the client
    c. Wash your hands on entering and leaving the room
    d. All of the above
29. Safety measures in the home include all of the following EXCEPT:
    a. Keeping the client's call bell within reach
    b. Wiping up spills as soon as possible
    c. Keeping the client's bed in the high position
    d. Locking the wheels on beds and wheelchairs when transferring clients
30. If you find yourself in an area filled with smoke:
    a. Cover your face with a damp cloth or towel
    b. Quickly open all windows and doors
    c. Run out of the area
    d. All of the above
31. When washing dishes, be sure to:
    a. Start with pots and pans first
    b. Rinse the dishes with cold water
    c. Allow washed items to air dry
    d. Wash dishes used by clients with infections first
32. Routine bathroom cleaning includes all of the following EXCEPT:
    a. Washing the bathroom window
    b. Cleaning the toilet bowl, seat, and outside areas
    c. Scrubbing the sink
    d. Mopping the floor
33. Daily cleaning of the client's room includes:
    a. Changing bed linens
    b. Dusting the furniture
    c. Disinfecting the bedframe
    d. All of the above

34. When ironing, it is best to:
    a. Iron items that require the highest heat setting first
    b. Have the clothes completely dry before ironing
    c. Check the care label for the correct iron setting
    d. Leave permanent press items in the dryer until ready to iron

35. All of the following are examples of good body mechanics EXCEPT:
    a. Standing with feet about 12 inches apart
    b. Bending from the waist to lift a heavy object
    c. Turning the whole body when changing directions, without twisting the back or neck
    d. Facing the work area

36. The client who is in the dorsal recumbent or back-lying position is in the:
    a. Supine position
    b. Lateral position
    c. Prone position
    d. Fowler's position

37. A client is correctly positioned in a chair if:
    a. The back of the knees touch the edge of the seat
    b. The back and buttocks are slightly away from the back of the chair
    c. The back of the knees and the calves are slightly away from the edge of the seat
    d. The feet do not touch the floor

38. Your client is a paraplegic. This means there is:
    a. Weakness on one side of the body
    b. Loss of sensation on one side of the body
    c. Loss of sensation and muscle function from the waist down
    d. Loss of sensation and muscle function from the neck down

39. When transferring a client from a bed to a wheelchair, be sure to:
    a. Have the client wear street shoes
    b. Help the client out of bed on his or her weak side
    c. Lower the footrests on the wheelchair
    d. Place the wheelchair at the foot of the bed

40. A four-point walking aid that is picked up and moved about 6 inches in front of the client is called:
    a. A cane
    b. A walker
    c. Crutches
    d. A brace

FINAL EXAMINATION

41. A supportive device used to prevent the hips and legs from turning outward is a:
    a. Handroll
    b. Bed cradle
    c. Footboard
    d. Trochanter roll

42. Straightening a body part is called:
    a. Flexion
    b. Extension
    c. Dorsiflexion
    d. Adduction

43. When performing range of motion exercises with a client, it is important to:
    a. Exercise all the joints of the body
    b. Do the exercises once a day
    c. Repeat each exercise two times
    d. Move the joint slowly, smoothly, and gently

44. A bed that is made while the client remains in it is called a/an:
    a. Occupied bed
    b. Hospital bed
    c. Closed bed
    d. Open bed

45. Some bed linen may be reused if it is not wet, soiled, or very wrinkled. One piece of linen that cannot be reused is the:
    a. Mattress pad
    b. Pillowcase
    c. Plastic drawsheet
    d. Bedspread

46. A glass thermometer has a red top and a round bulb. It is used for:
    a. Axillary temperatures
    b. Oral temperatures
    c. A child's temperature
    d. Rectal temperatures

47. Clean a glass thermometer in:
    a. Cold, soapy water
    b. Warm, soapy water
    c. Alcohol
    d. Hot, running water

48. An oral thermometer needs to remain in the client's mouth:
    a. 5 minutes
    b. 8 to 9 minutes
    c. 3 to 4 minutes
    d. 10 to 11 minutes

49. The most frequently used pulse point is the:
    a. Apical
    b. Radial
    c. Carotid
    d. Brachial
50. These statements are about taking a radial pulse. Which one is FALSE?
    a. The radial artery is located on the thumb side of the wrist.
    b. The thumb is used to feel the pulse.
    c. The pulse is counted for 30 seconds, then the number is multiplied by 2.
    d. The client should sit or lie down.
51. Mr. K. is having respirations that are very rapid and deep. This is an example of:
    a. Apnea
    b. Cheyne-Stokes
    c. Orthopnea
    d. Hyperventilation
52. A client is having bradypnea if:
    a. Respirations are more than 24 per minute
    b. Respirations are less than 10 per minute
    c. The abdomen rather than the chest rises and falls
    d. No respirations are being taken
53. The artery that is normally used to measure blood pressure is the:
    a. Radial
    b. Brachial
    c. Carotid
    d. Femoral
54. Which statement is FALSE about blood pressure measurement?
    a. The blood pressure is not taken in an arm with an IV.
    b. The client needs to rest about 15 minutes before taking the blood pressure.
    c. Blood pressure cuffs are not applied over clothing.
    d. The blood pressure cuff should be wide enough to cover about half of the upper arm.
55. Inflate the blood pressure cuff:
    a. To 200 mm Hg for all clients
    b. 30 mm Hg beyond the point where you last felt the radial pulse
    c. 30 mm Hg beyond the point where you last heard the client's blood pressure
    d. 15 mm Hg beyond the point where you last felt the radial pulse

56. Your client's blood pressure is 178/70. You would know:
    a. That this is a normal blood pressure
    b. The systolic pressure is above normal
    c. The diastolic pressure is above normal
    d. The client has hypotension
57. Which of these children should NOT have a rectal temperature taken?
    a. An 8-month-old infant
    b. A 3-year-old child with a history of seizures
    c. A 4-year-old boy with diarrhea
    d. A newborn infant
58. Which temperature reading should be reported immediately?
    a. Rectal temperature of 99.6° F.
    b. Oral temperature of 37° C.
    c. Axillary temperature of 97.2° F.
    d. Rectal temperature of 38.8° C.
59. Providing mouth care for the unconscious client would include all EXCEPT:
    a. Positioning the client on one side with the head turned well to the side
    b. Using lemon glycerine swabs for all mouth care
    c. Keeping the client's mouth open with the use of a padded tongue blade
    d. Using very small amounts of fluid
60. Dentures need to be cleaned:
    a. Whenever the client requests it
    b. Once each day
    c. When the client goes to sleep
    d. As often as natural teeth
61. Which statement about denture care is FALSE?
    a. Gloves should be worn during this procedure.
    b. Dentures should be removed by using gauze to grasp the upper denture first, then remove the lower.
    c. Denture cleaner or toothpaste is used to brush the dentures.
    d. Rinse the dentures under hot running water in a sink lined with a towel.
62. You are about to give your client a complete bed bath. You should FIRST:
    a. Gather all supplies
    b. Wash your hands
    c. Offer the bedpan or urinal
    d. Explain what you are going to do

63. In a partial bath, the client washes:
    a. All areas except the perineal area
    b. All areas except the back
    c. All areas that can be easily reached
    d. The face, hands, and chest
64. All are true about assisting a client with a tub bath EXCEPT:
    a. Place a rubber mat on the bottom of the tub and a bath mat on the floor in front
    b. Fill the tub halfway with 105° F water
    c. Do not disturb the client while he or she is in the tub
    d. Clean the tub before and after use
65. A back massage is ended with:
    a. Long, firm stokes
    b. Circular motions with the tips of your fingers
    c. Fast, choppy strokes
    d. Kneading tissue between the thumb and fingers
66. Which statement about perineal care is FALSE?
    a. Work from the cleanest area to the dirtiest.
    b. Clean the anal area last.
    c. Use warm water and wear disposable gloves.
    d. Do not use soap.
67. All of these measures help prevent decubitus ulcers EXCEPT:
    a. Vigorous rubbing of the skin
    b. Repositioning the client every two hours
    c. Keeping the skin clean especially of urine and feces
    d. Using lotion on dry areas and powder between skin areas that touch
68. Clients at risk of developing bedsores include those:
    a. Who are inactive and bedridden
    b. With poor circulation
    c. Unable to control bowels and bladders
    d. All of the above
69. Which statement is TRUE regarding dressing the client with an IV?
    a. Dress the side with the IV first
    b. Dress the strong arm first
    c. Remove the garment from the arm with the IV first
    d. Do not remove the IV bottle from the pole at any time
70. The main goal for clients with indwelling catheters is to:
    a. Keep the client dry
    b. Prevent infection
    c. Gain bladder control
    d. Increase the amount of urine produced

71. Which of the following does NOT need to be reported to the nurse about a client with an indwelling catheter?
    a. The client feels a strong urge to urinate.
    b. The urine is leaking around the catheter.
    c. The urine is amber and has a faint odor.
    d. The client has a discharge from the penis.
72. For catheter care, it is important to:
    a. Wear gloves and protect the client's privacy
    b. Clean from about 4 inches down the catheter to the meatus
    c. Use the same cotton ball or gauze pad for each stroke
    d. Do all of the above
73. Leg bags are used for:
    a. Male clients
    b. Clients who have little urine output
    c. Clients confined to bed
    d. Clients who are up and about
74. Which observation needs to be reported to the nurse?
    a. Your client has liquid brown stools every two hours.
    b. Your client's abdomen is soft and flat.
    c. The stool of your client is soft-formed and brown.
    d. Your client has a bowel movement every morning.
75. In collecting any urine specimen, it is important to do all EXCEPT:
    a. Collect the first urine of the morning
    b. Wear gloves to avoid contact with the urine
    c. Ask the client not to have a bowel movement while the urine is being collected
    d. Label the specimen with the client's name, address, date and time, and type of specimen
76. For a mid-stream urine sample:
    a. All urine is collected for 24 hours
    b. The client voids once, discards that urine, then voids again in 30 minutes
    c. The perineal area is cleaned before the urine is collected
    d. The urine must be passed through a 4 x 4 gauze
77. Which is the most balanced meal?
    a. Hamburger on a bun, potato chips, coffee
    b. Tuna salad on whole wheat bread, milk
    c. Cheese pizza, diet soda
    d. Macaroni and cheese, Polish sausage, milk

78. You are to prepare a meal for a client who is on a low-sodium diet. Which food should be avoided?
    a. Carrots
    b. Canned spaghetti sauce
    c. Chicken
    d. Peaches
79. When feeding a client, it is best to:
    a. Serve foods in the order preferred by the client
    b. Offer the solid foods first, followed by the liquids
    c. Use a fork except for semi-liquid foods
    d. Keep conversation to a minimum to encourage the client to eat
80. Your client is on Intake and Output. He just drank 4 ounces of juice. You would record:
    a. 4 ounces liquid
    b. 4 ounces oral intake
    c. 120 ml oral intake
    d. 400 cc oral intake
81. You are assisting your client with her medication. It is acceptable for you to do all of the following EXCEPT:
    a. Read the medication label carefully
    b. Know how much of the drug the client must take
    c. Keep all the medicines for the client in one container
    d. Offer water or other liquid to help the client swallow the medicine
82. An ice collar is ordered for your client. Which statement is FALSE?
    a. Replace the cover if it becomes wet.
    b. Keep the collar in place for 30 minutes.
    c. Fill the collar with crushed ice.
    d. Check the skin every 15 minutes for complications.
83. Leg exercises done after surgery are helpful in preventing a thrombus, which is a/an:
    a. Blood clot
    b. Infection in the lung
    c. Collapse of the lung
    d. Blood clot that lodges in the lungs
84. Which statement about breast-feeding is FALSE?
    a. Breast-fed infants may need to nurse every two to three hours.
    b. Mothers should nurse from both breasts at each feeding.
    c. Nursing mothers will need more calories and fluids in their diets.
    d. Burping is not necessary in babies who are breast-fed.

85. Which statement about bottle feeding is FALSE?
    a. Bottles of formula should be warmed before feeding.
    b. Plastic nursers do not have to be sterilized.
    c. Burp the baby when about half of the formula has been taken.
    d. Refrigerate any formula remaining in the bottle.
86. Umbilical cord care is done:
    a. Once a day
    b. Until the cord stump comes off
    c. With alcohol at each diaper change
    d. Only if an infection is present
87. You are giving a baby a sponge bath. The first area of the body to clean would be the:
    a. Face
    b. Eyes
    c. Nose
    d. Ears
88. Your client has suffered a broken bone in which the bone came through the skin. This is a:
    a. Simple fracture
    b. Closed fracture
    c. Compound fracture
    d. Reduced fracture
89. Your client has suffered a stroke. Which of the following will help prevent contractures?
    a. Frequent turning and repositioning
    b. Bladder training
    c. Elastic stockings
    d. Range-of-motion exercises
90. All of these measures are helpful when caring for the blind person EXCEPT:
    a. Identifying yourself promptly and before touching the person
    b. Keeping furniture and equipment in an arrangement familiar to the client
    c. Leaving doors partly open
    d. Warning the client of steps, turns, curbs, and other hazards when ambulating
91. The client with emphysema will usually prefer to:
    a. Be in the side-lying position
    b. Sit upright and slightly forward
    c. Be in semi-Fowler's position
    d. Keep the head of the bed flat

92. Your client is a diabetic. It is important to
    a. Provide excellent skin care, especially to the feet
    b. Prepare meals according to the diet plan and serve them on time
    c. Test the client's urine as directed
    d. Do all of the above

93. In an emergency situation, do all of the following EXCEPT:
    a. Stay calm and help the victim feel more secure
    b. Keep the victim lying down or in the position in which he or she was found
    c. Try to get the conscious victim to drink water
    d. Keep the victim warm

94. Which is NOT a sign of cardiac arrest?
    a. Low blood pressure
    b. No pulse
    c. No respirations
    d. Skin is cool, pale, and gray

95. You find a client unconscious on the floor in her apartment. Your first action would be to:
    a. Call your supervisor
    b. Check for breathing, a pulse, and bleeding
    c. Call for help
    d. Perform CPR

96. Your client suddenly has a grand mal seizure. It is important to do all of these actions EXCEPT:
    a. Lower the client to the floor
    b. Protect the head with a blanket, a pillow, or cradle it in your lap
    c. Loosen tight clothing, such as ties or shirt collars
    d. Restrain the client's movements as much as possible

97. You walk into a room and find that a 2-year-old child has been drinking bleach. Your first action is to:
    a. Activate the EMS system
    b. Maintain an open airway; give CPR if necessary
    c. Make the child vomit
    d. Call your supervisor

98. First aid for a burn is:
    a. Applying a cream for burns
    b. Packing the burn in ice
    c. Pouring cool water over the burned area
    d. Covering the burned area with a wet dressing

99. As death approaches:
    a. Movement, muscle tone, and sensation are lost
    b. Body temperature falls
    c. Blood pressure rises
    d. Pain increases
100. A living will insures that:
    a. Every effort will be made to prolong life
    b. No heroic measures will be used to prolong life
    c. The client will die at home
    d. CPR will be attempted

Answers to Chapter Questions

CHAPTER 1: Introduction to Home Care

TERMS TO KNOW

1. Medicare
2. plan of treatment
3. homebound
4. hospice
5. diagnostic related groups
6. Medicaid
7. health maintenance organization
8. homemaker
9. home health aide
10. policy and procedure manual

TRUE AND FALSE

1. F — less expensive
2. T
3. F — homemaker services
4. F — Medicare
5. T
6. F — nursing policies and procedures
7. T
8. T
9. F — your supervisor
10. T

MULTIPLE CHOICE

1. terminal
2. organizational chart
3. registered nurse
4. doctor
5. physical therapist
6. social worker
7. HMO

ANSWERS TO CHAPTER QUESTIONS

CROSSWORD PUZZLE

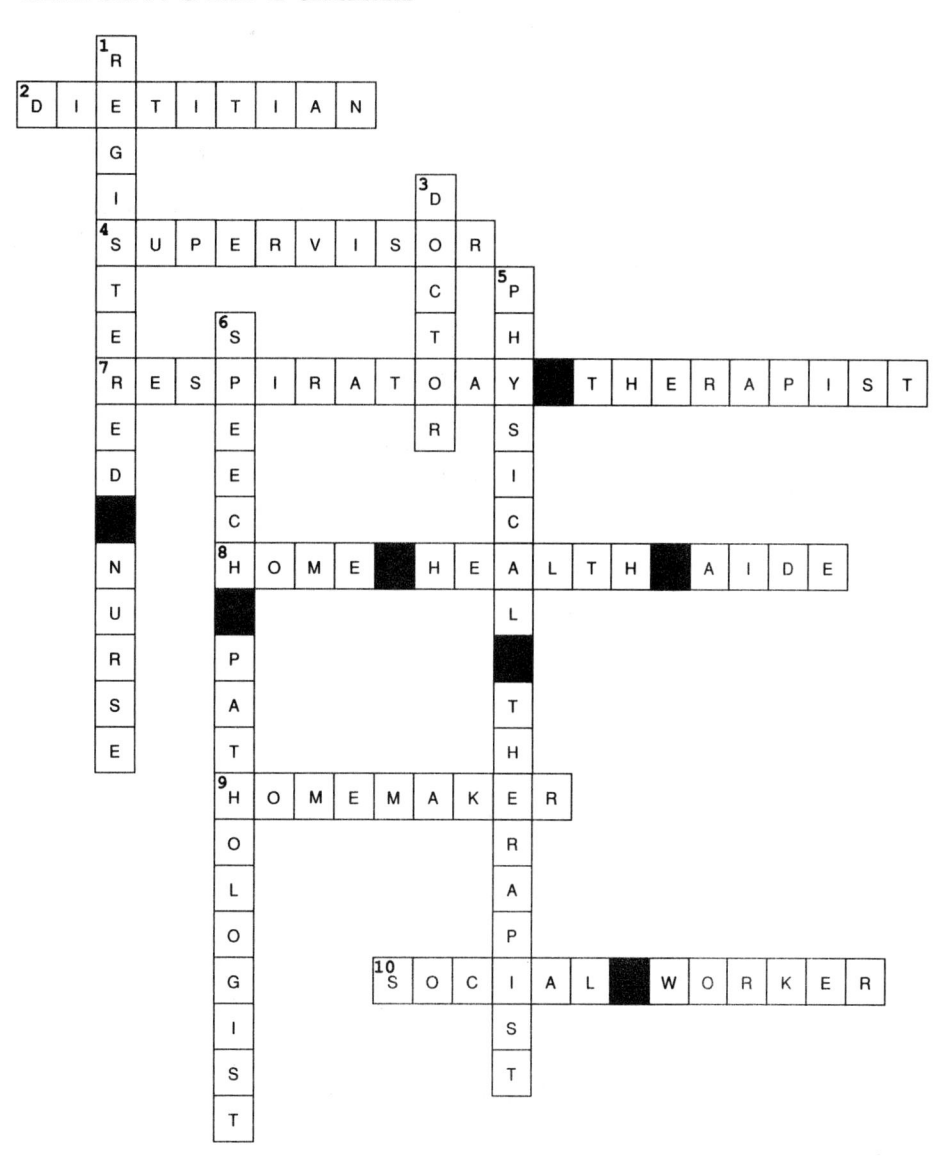

(Across): 2. DIETITIAN, 4. SUPERVISOR, 7. RESPIRATORY THERAPIST, 8. HOME HEALTH AIDE, 9. HOMEMAKER, 10. SOCIAL WORKER

(Down): 1. REGISTERED NURSE, 3. DOCTOR, 5. PHYSICIST, 6. SPEECH PATHOLOGIST, (additional) PHYSICAL THERAPIST

CHAPTER 2: The Home Health Aide

TERMS TO KNOW

1. c
2. f
3. d
4. b
5. g
6. a
7. h
8. e

UNDERSTANDING ROLES AND RESPONSIBILITIES

1. yes
2. yes
3. no
4. yes
5. yes
6. no
7. yes
8. no
9. yes
10. no
11. no
12. no

TRUE AND FALSE

1. F — not to have
2. T
3. T
4. F — before
5. F — negligence
6. T
7. F — client, the family or employee
8. F — report it immediately
9. T
10. F — You may not

MULTIPLE CHOICE

1. sensitivity
2. conscientiousness
3. may not
4. your supervisor
5. wedding rings
6. battery
7. false imprisonment
8. Many
9. do not
10. cannot

LIST

1. a. How will my behavior affect the client?
   b. How will my behavior affect the family?
   c. How will my behavior affect my employer?
   d. How will my behavior affect me?
2. Any two of the following: refusing to care for a client because of race, religion, age, or moral beliefs; rudeness; unreliable; dishonesty; stealing; ridiculing; gossiping; sexual contact; sharing confidential information.
3. Any two of the following: failure to report changes in client's condition; leaving a home before relief person arrives; damage to property; unsafe practices resulting in client injury.
4. Any two of the following: client falls; burns to you or the client; client accuses you of stealing; you injure yourself in the client's home.

CHAPTER 3: Communicating Effectively
TERMS TO KNOW
1. communication
2. body language
3. cliche
4. nonverbal communication
5. Verbal communication
6. tact
7. feedback

TRUE AND FALSE
1. F — nonverbal
2. T
3. F — nonverbal
4. T
5. F — is very different than
6. T
7. F — tell your supervisor
8. T
9. F — does not improve
10. F — with your supervisor

COMMUNICATING EFFECTIVELY
Items to be checked: 1, 5, 7, 8, 10, 11
Communication barriers:
3. Changing the subject
4. Giving opinions or advice
9. Lack of trust (not being honest) or cliches

CHAPTER 4: Communicating in the Home Health Agency
TERMS TO KNOW
1. d
2. g
3. e
4. h
5. f
6. c
7. b
8. a

FORMING MEDICAL TERMS
1. dyspnea
2. intravenous
3. hyperthyroid
4. tachycardia
5. polyuria
6. transabdominal
7. endocardial
8. hepatomegaly
9. pharyngitis
10. mastectomy
11. neuroma
12. cephalgia
13. hemorrhage
14. gastrostomy
15. rhinoplasty
16. bronchoscopy

CLIENT RECORDS

1. f
2. h
3. a
4. c
5. g
6. e
7. b
8. h
9. d
10. a
11. e
12. g

MULTIPLE CHOICE

1. sign
2. subjective
3. black ink
4. two
5. giving personal care
6. use quotation marks
7. was not
8. draw a line through the wrong entry and write "error"
9. may not
10. avoid

MATCHING

Part 1.

1. e
2. g
3. f
4. c
5. j
6. d
7. i
8. b
9. h
10. a

Part 2.

11. d
12. i
13. g
14. b
15. k
16. c
17. l
18. j
19. f
20. h
21. a
22. e

ANSWERS TO CHAPTER QUESTIONS

CROSSWORD PUZZLE

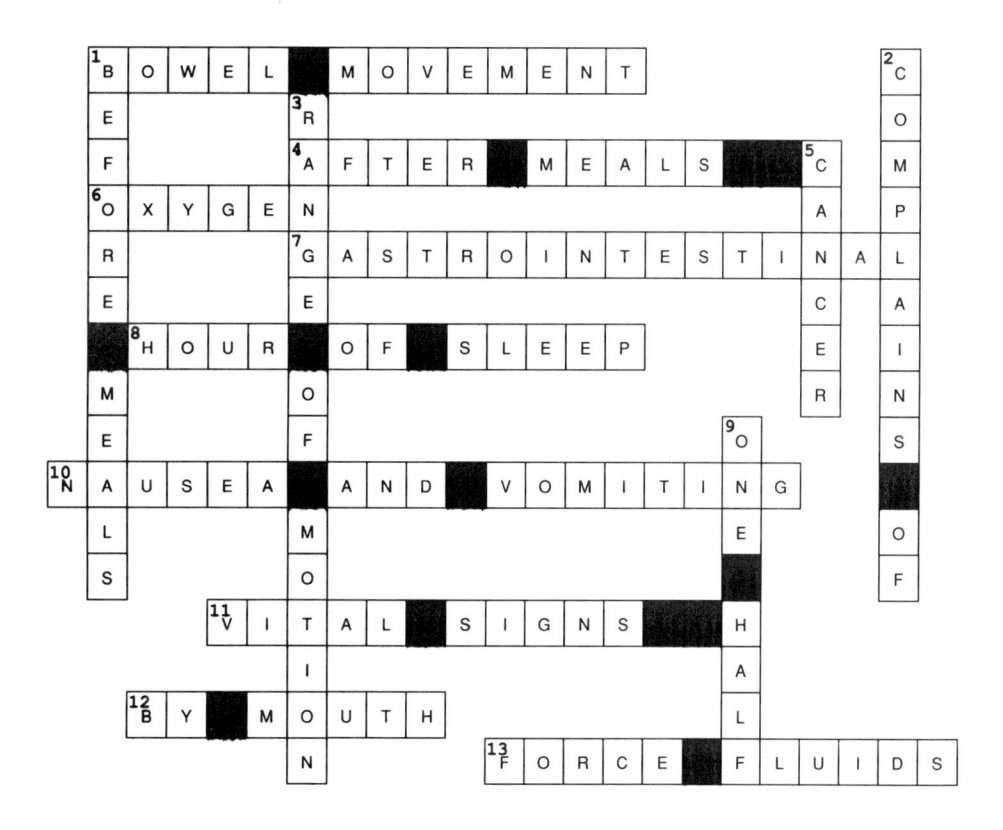

	1	2	3	4	5	6	7	8	9	10	11	12	13	14
1	B	O	W	E	L		M	O	V	E	M	E	N	T
	E						R							C
	F				A	F	T	E	R		M	E	A	L	S		C	O
	O	X	Y	G	E	N								A
	R				G	A	S	T	R	O	I	N	T	E	S	T	I	N	A	L
	E				E									C
		H	O	U	R		O	F		S	L	E	E	P
	M				O									R
	E				F					O				N	S
	N	A	U	S	E	A		A	N	D		V	O	M	I	T	I	N	G
	L				M					E				O
	S				O									F
					V	I	T	A	L		S	I	G	N	S		H
					I									A
		B	Y		M	O	U	T	H					L
					N					F	O	R	C	E		F	L	U	I	D	S

(Crossword grid — layout reproduced approximately)

CHAPTER 5: Understanding the Needs of Clients

TERMS TO KNOW

1. disability
2. menopause
3. sexuality
4. need
5. self-esteem
6. extended family
7. puberty
8. menarche
9. bias
10. esteem
11. culture
12. nuclear family
13. aging

TRUE AND FALSE

1. T
2. F — need for love and belonging
3. T
4. F — Adolescence
5. T
6. T
7. F — decrease
8. F — very rapidly
9. T
10. T

GROWTH AND DEVELOPMENT

1. g	6. h	11. a
2. c	7. b	12. c
3. a	8. e	13. e
4. d	9. b	14. f
5. f	10. e	15. d

FILL IN

Stage	Age	Examples of Toy/Activity For Age
Infancy	*0–1*	*Rattles, soft animals, big balls*
Toddler	*1–3*	*Push–pull toys, play dough, books*
Preschool	*3–6*	Puzzles, trucks, dolls, tricycles
School age	*6–12*	*Crafts, group activities, sports*
Adolescence	*12–18*	*Music, dances, talking on phone*

MULTIPLE CHOICE

1. infancy
2. school
3. school
4. less
5. preschool
6. menopause
7. birth

CHAPTER 6: Understanding How the Body Functions

TERMS TO KNOW

Part 1.
1. d
2. f
3. a
4. b
5. c
6. e

Part 2.
1. c
2. d
3. e
4. a

5. f
6. b

Part 3.
1. c
2. e
3. f
4. a
5. d
6. b

Part 4.
1. c
2. d

3. e
4. a
5. b

Part 5.
1. c
2. f
3. a
4. b
5. g
6. e
7. d

ANSWERS TO CHAPTER QUESTIONS

MULTIPLE CHOICE

1. epithelial
2. organs
3. dermis
4. dilate
5. long
6. joint
7. Cartilage
8. smooth
9. tendons
10. contraction
11. cerebral cortex
12. pupil
13. eustachian tube
14. inner
15. red blood cells
16. atria
17. aorta
18. poor
19. larynx
20. alveoli
21. stomach
22. small
23. bladder
24. testosterone
25. cervix
26. menstruation
27. pituitary
28. thyroid
29. pancreas
30. pituitary

FILL IN

1. a. covers and protects the body
   b. senses heat, cold, pain, and pressure
   c. helps control body temperature
2. a. long bones; Example: leg and arm bones
   b. short bones; Example: wrist, fingers, ankles, toes
   c. flat bones; Example: rib, pelvic, and skull
   d. irregular bones; Example: vertebrae
3. a. move body parts
   b. maintain posture
   c. produce body heat
4. a. center of thought and intelligence
   b. regulates and coordinates body movements
   c. controls heart rate, breathing, blood vessel size, swallowing, coughing, and vomiting
5. a. eye
   b. ear
   c. nose
   d. tongue
   e. skin
6. a. transport oxygen and carbon dioxide through bloodstream
   b. protect the body against infection
   c. needed for blood clotting

7. a. nose
   b. pharynx
   c. larynx
   d. trachea
   e. bronchus
8. a. duodenum
   b. jejunum
   c. ileum
9. a. kidney
   b. ureter
   c. bladder
   d. urethra
10. a. produce male sex cells and testosterone
    b. store sperm and produce semen
    c. secretes a fluid into semen
    d. produce female sex cells and female hormones
    e. transports ova (egg) from ovary to uterus
    f. provides a place for fetus to grow and be nourished
    g. receives the penis during intercourse; birth canal
    h. secrete milk after childbirth

LABELING

FIG. 6–1. The brain.

a. cerebrum
b. cerebellum
c. brainstem

FIG. 6–2. The heart.

1. superior vena cava
2. aorta
3. right atrium
4. right ventricle
5. left atrium
6. left ventricle

FIG. 6–3. The respiratory system.

1. pharynx
2. trachea
3. right main bronchus
4. bronchiole
5. pleura
6. left main bronchus
7. alveolus

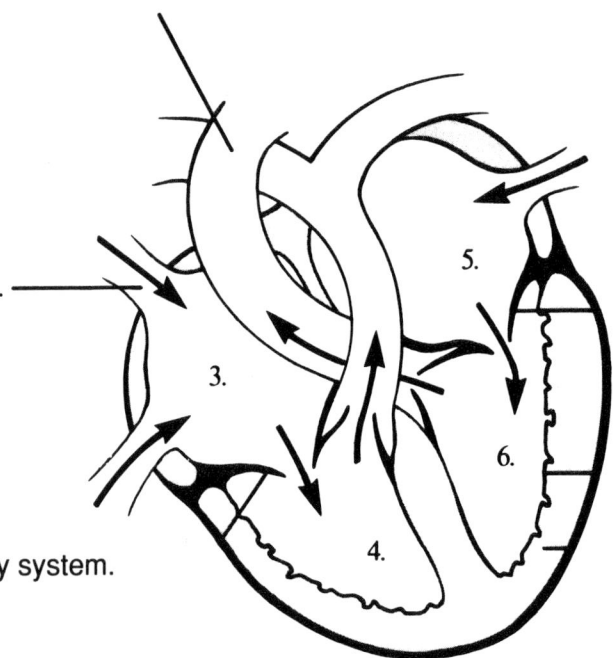

ANSWERS TO CHAPTER QUESTIONS

FIG. 6–4. The digestive system.

1. mouth
2. pharynx
3. esophagus
4. liver
5. gallbladder
6. small intestine
7. anus
8. stomach
9. pancreas
10. large intestine
11. rectum

FIG. 6–5. The urinary system.

1. kidney
2. ureter
3. bladder
4. urethra

FIG. 6–6. The male reproductive system.

1. urinary bladder
2. vas deferens
3. prostate gland
4. rectum
5. ejaculatory duct
6. epididymis
7. testicle
8. penis
9. scrotum

FIG. 6–7. The female reproductive system.

1. fallopian tube
2. ovary
3. uterus
4. external genitalia
5. vagina
6. cervix

WORD ASSOCIATION

1. large intestine
2. tympanic membrane
3. cerumen
4. pharynx
5. larynx
6. sclera
7. trachea
8. uterus

CHAPTER 7: Controlling Infection in the Home
TERMS TO KNOW

1. sterilization
2. pathogen
3. Contamination
4. asepsis
5. clean technique
6. microorganism
7. disinfection
8. medical asepsis
9. nonpathogen
10. infection
11. sterile

TRUE AND FALSE

1. F — moist
2. F — will not kill; will slow the growth of
3. T
4. F — is not the same
5. T
6. F — dirty
7. F — away from
8. F — from the cleanest to the dirtiest
9. T
10. T
11. F — cold water
12. F — will not
13. T
14. F — two persons
15. T

CHECKING UP ON PROCEDURES

Handwashing: 4, 2, 6, 1, 5, 3
Wet Heat Sterilization: 3, 2, 1, 4

MULTIPLE CHOICE

1. 15
2. heat
3. 20
4. clean
5. gloves-gown-mask
6. spores
7. wet
8. ties
9. dry
10. before

MATCHING

1. c
2. b
3. d
4. a
5. e

ANSWERS TO CHAPTER QUESTIONS

LIST

1. a. host
   b. water
   c. warmth
   d. oxygen
   e. darkness
   f. food
2. Any six of the following: fever, pain or tenderness, fatigue, loss of appetite, nausea, vomiting, diarrhea, rash, sores on mucous membranes, redness and swelling of a body part, discharge or drainage from an area
3. a. SOAP — bar or liquid from a dispenser
   b. WATER — clean, warm, running water
   c. FRICTION — rubbing the hands together

CHAPTER 8: Safety

TRUE AND FALSE

1. T
2. F — Falls
3. F — in bedrooms and bathrooms
4. F — should be locked
5. T
6. F — turned off
7. T
8. F — bottom
9. F — even if it is (you call for them)
10. T

MULTIPLE CHOICE

1. the elderly
2. low
3. cotton
4. close
5. good
6. before
7. the nearest police or gas station
8. the driver
9. facing you
10. do not go

CHECKING UP ON PROCEDURES

Using a Fire Extinguisher: 3, 2, 5, 4, 1

SAFE OR UNSAFE?

1. S
2. U — Your action is safe, but not enough. You must have the odor promptly investigated by competent repairmen.
3. U — The cord should be repaired by someone trained to do electrical work.
4. S
5. U — Having such a list is excellent. Put it by the phone.
6. S
7. U — With poor vision, the client may easily reach for the wrong medicine. Put the medicine in a safe, locked area and bring it to him at the correct time.
8. S
9. S
10. U — You might forget to follow through. Change the bulb immediately.

HIDDEN WORD SEARCH

1. F(A)L L
2. (C)O M A
3. S U F F O(C)A T I O N
4. F(I)R E
5. G R O U N(D)
6. O X Y G(E)N
7. B U R(N)S
8. I N F E C(T)I O N
9. P O I(S)O N I N G

Hidden Word: ACCIDENTS

CHAPTER 9: Home Maintenance

TERMS TO KNOW

1. d
2. c
3. e
4. a
5. f
6. g
7. b

ANSWERS TO CHAPTER QUESTIONS

TRUE AND FALSE
1. T
2. F — Client care
3. F — cleaned with a spray-on foam
4. F — do not mix
5. T
6. F — as soon as possible
7. T
8. F — Machine washing cleans and disinfects better
9. F — Dampen clothing
10. T

MULTIPLE CHOICE
1. specialty cleaner
2. 15 minutes
3. 3 days
4. hot
5. cleanest
6. should not
7. air
8. daily
9. cold
10. prewash product

MATCHING
1. W
2. D
3. W
4. A
5. D
6. A
7. D
8. W, A
9. A
10. D
11. D
12. A
13. W
14. D
15. W

CHAPTER 10: Body Mechanics
TERMS TO KNOW
Part 1.
1. d
2. e
3. b
4. c
5. a

Part 2.
1. e
2. d
3. f
4. g
5. b
6. c
7. a

LABELING
Fig. 10–1. Supine

Fig. 10–2. Prone

Fig. 10–3. Sims'

Fig. 10–4. Lateral

Fig. 10–5. Fowler's

TRUE AND FALSE

1. F — shoulders, upper arms, hips and thighs
2. T
3. F — supine position is the same as
4. T
5. T
6. F — as much as possible
7. T
8. F — off-center or in the back
9. F — do not have; hold the straps or chains
10. T

CHECKING UP ON PROCEDURES

Moving the Client Up in Bed with Client's Help: 5, 2, 4, 1, 3
Moving the Client to the Side of the Bed: 3, 5, 2, 1, 4
Transferring the Client to a Chair/Wheelchair: 3, 5, 1, 4, 2, 6
Protecting the Client During a Fall: 2, 4, 5, 6, 1, 3

MULTIPLE CHOICE

1. wide
2. up
3. 45 to 60 degrees
4. slightly away from
5. Rolling
6. stop immediately
7. over
8. strong
9. call an ambulance
10. warm

CHAPTER 11: Activity

TERMS TO KNOW

1. prosthesis
2. embolus
3. footdrop
4. activities of daily living
5. atrophy
6. range of motion
7. thrombus
8. rehabilitation
9. contracture
10. plantar flexion

TRUE AND FALSE

1. T
2. F — weak side
3. F — physical therapist or nurse will teach
4. F — may be attached
5. T
6. F — not the same (although both items will keep linens off the client's feet)
7. T
8. T
9. T
10. F — five to six times per jointl
11. T

ANSWERS TO CHAPTER QUESTIONS

MULTIPLE CHOICE

1. well-fitting
2. strong
3. weak
4. decrease
5. rolled washcloths
6. passive
7. supine
8. neck
9. artificial eye
10. abilities

CHECKING UP ON PROCEDURES

Helping the Client Walk: 3, 1, 5, 2, 4, 6

MATCHING

1. d
2. g
3. e
4. h
5. c
6. j
7. b
8. i
9. k
10. a
11. f

CROSSWORD PUZZLE

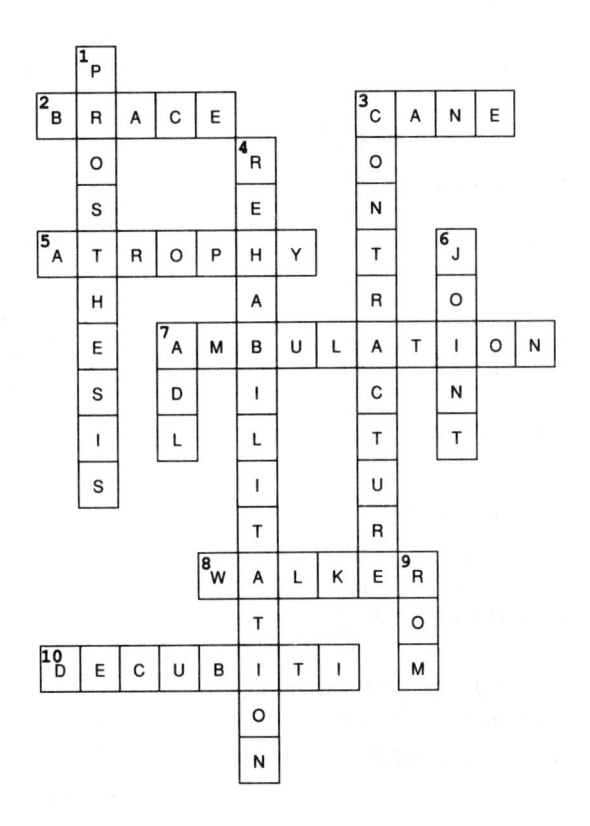

			¹P						
²B	R	A	C	E		³C	A	N	E
	O			⁴R		O			
	S			E		N			
⁵A	T	R	O	P	H	Y		⁶J	
	H			A		R		O	
	E	⁷A	M	B	U	L	A	T	I	O	N
	S	D		I		C		N	
	I	L		L		T		T	
	S			I		U			
				T		R			
			⁸W	A	L	K	E	⁹R	
				T				O	
¹⁰D	E	C	U	B	I	T	I		M
						O			
						N			

CHAPTER 12: Bedmaking

TERMS TO KNOW

1. mitered corner
2. Trendelenburg's
3. occupied bed
4. drawsheet
5. closed bed
6. open bed
7. Fowler's
8. plastic drawsheet
9. Semi-Fowler's

TRUE AND FALSE

1. T
2. F — down position
3. F — semi-Fowler's position (head is also raised 45 degrees)
4. T
5. F — should never be placed
6. F — cotton drawsheet must be used with a plastic
7. T
8. T
9. F — 14 inches
10. T

LABELING

FIG. 12–1.
a. raises the bed horizontally
b. raises head of bed
c. raises knee portion

FIG. 12–2.
a. old cotton drawsheet
b. old plastic drawsheet
c. old bottom sheet
d. clean bottom sheet
e. clean cotton drawsheet
f. clean plastic drawsheet

MULTIPLE CHOICE

1. once a week
2. away from
3. toward
4. plastic drawsheet
5. disposable bed protectors
6. mended
7. pillowcase
8. be tucked in together
9. away from
10. before

ANSWERS TO CHAPTER QUESTIONS

CHAPTER 13: Vital Signs

TERMS TO KNOW

1. e
2. h
3. f
4. j
5. g
6. b
7. i
8. a
9. d
10. c

TRUE AND FALSE

1. F — as often as you are instructed
2. F — do not need to report; you do need to record . . . even if they are . . .
3. T
4. F — should be taken
5. F — 60 to 100
6. T
7. F — may not be
8. F — at the level of the heart
9. T
10. T

MULTIPLE CHOICE

1. morning
2. change
3. constantly
4. 98.6° F
5. Axillary
6. round and stubby
7. stem to the bulb
8. cold
9. 15
10. axillary
11. apical
12. 1 minute
13. left
14. alcohol wipes
15. Do not tell
16. hypertension
17. aneroid
18. two-thirds
19. systolic
20. 3

CHECKING UP ON PROCEDURES

Measuring a Rectal Temperature: 2, 6, 1, 7, 5, 3, 4
Taking a Radial Pulse: 4, 3, 6, 1, 2, 5
Taking an Apical Pulse: 3, 1, 4, 5, 2
Taking a Blood Pressure: 4, 3, 5, 1, 2, 6, 7

READING THERMOMETERS

FIG. 13–1. 99.4° F = 37.4° C
FIG. 13–2. 100.8° F = 38.2° C
FIG. 13–3. 102.6° F = 39.2° C
FIG. 13–4. 101° F = 38.3° C
FIG. 13–5. 104.4° F = 40.2° C

CHARTING VITAL SIGNS

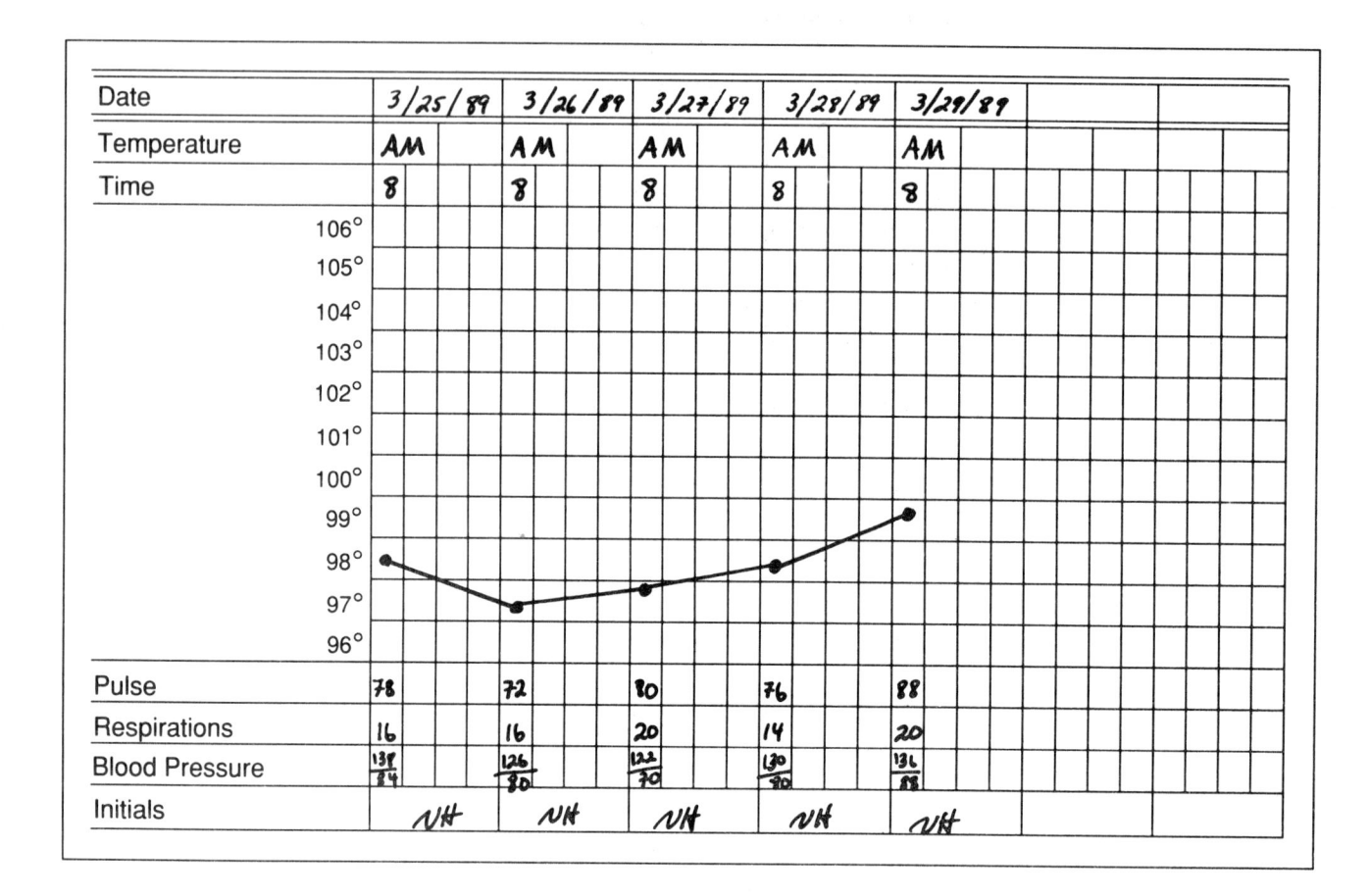

Date	3/25/89	3/26/89	3/27/89	3/28/89	3/29/89			
Temperature	AM	AM	AM	AM	AM			
Time	8	8	8	8	8			
Temperature (°F)	98°	97°	97.5°	98°	99°			
Pulse	78	72	80	76	88			
Respirations	16	16	20	14	20			
Blood Pressure	138/84	126/80	122/70	130/80	136/88			
Initials	NH	NH	NH	NH	NH			

ANSWERS TO CHAPTER QUESTIONS

LIST

1. a. has fallen or been injured
   b. complains of feeling ill
   c. shows signs of illness
   d. shows a change in behavior
   e. sudden change in condition
2. Any five of the following: age, sex, amount of blood in the system, emotions, body size, medications, exercise, pain, time of day, activity level
3. a. Oral: 97.6 to 99.6° F (36.5 to 37.5° C)
   b. Rectal: 98.6 to 100.6° F (37 to 38.1° C)
   c. Axillary: 96.6 to 98.6° F (36 to 37° C)
4. Any five of the following: temporal, carotid, brachial, radial, femoral, popliteal, dorsalis pedis (pedal), and apical

CROSSWORD PUZZLE

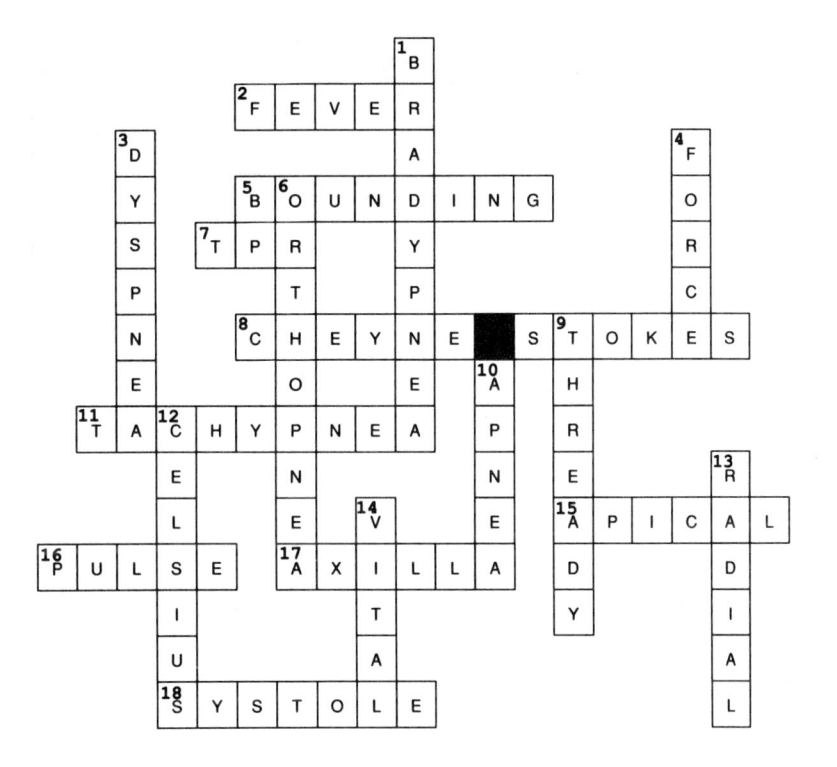

							1 B					
			2 F	E	V	E	R					
	3 D						A				4 F	
	Y		5 B	6 O	U	N	D	I	N	G	O	
	S	7 T	P	R			Y				R	
	P			T			P				C	
	N		8 C	H	E	Y	N	E		9 T	O	K	E	S
	E			O			E	10 A		H	
11 T	A	12 C	H	Y	P	N	E	A	P	R		13 R
		E			N			N	E		R
		L			E	14 V		E	15 A	P	I	C	A	L
16 P	U	L	S	E	17 A	X	I	L	L	A	D		D
		I				T			Y		I
		U				A					A
		18 S	Y	S	T	O	L	E			L

CHAPTER 14: Personal Care

TERMS TO KNOW

1. decubitus ulcer
2. deodorant
3. antiperspirant
4. perineal care
5. aspiration

TRUE AND FALSE

1. T
2. F — do as much as possible for himself/herself with
3. F — The client
4. F — It is necessary
5. T
6. F — Clients should
7. T
8. T
9. T
10. F — The nurse may change
11. T
12. T
13. F — as often as necessary (at least three times)
14. F — are not allowed
15. F — Leave the room only if the client is able to stand without help
16. T
17. F — genital and anal areas
18. T
19. F — Soak the hands before cutting the fingernails. (Home health aides do not cut toenails.)
20. F — is pale or white skin or a reddened area
21. T
22. F — Preventing skin from coming in contact with skin
23. F — circular motion
24. T
25. T

MULTIPLE CHOICE

1. maximum
2. soft
3. side-lying
4. at bedtime
5. 18 inches
6. upper right side
7. a padded tongue blade
8. back-and-forth
9. container filled with cool water
10. powder
11. 110 to 115° F
12. farthest
13. perineum
14. after
15. 20
16. 105
17. 4 to 6
18. anal
19. 2
20. stronger

MATCHING

1. c
2. f
3. b
4. e
5. a
6. d
7. g

ANSWERS TO CHAPTER QUESTIONS

CHECKING UP ON PROCEDURES

Providing Mouth Care for an Unconscious Client: 5, 4, 1, 6, 3, 2
Denture Care: 3, 5, 2, 1, 4
Giving a Partial Bath: 2, 6, 3, 4, 1, 5
Giving a Back Massage: 1, 6, 2, 4, 3, 5

LIST

1. Any five of the following: color of the skin, lips, nail beds, and sclera of the eyes; location and description of rashes; dry skin; bruises or open areas of the skin; pale or reddened areas, particularly over bony parts; drainage or bleeding from wounds or body openings; skin temperature; client complaints of pain or discomfort

2. Any five of the following: elderly; paralyzed; bedbound; obese; very thin; malnourished

Also, clients who cannot control their bowels and bladder; have a decreased ability to feel heat, cold, or pressure; are heavily sedated with medication; have poor circulation; are diabetic, have casts or who are in traction.

CHAPTER 15: Elimination

TERMS TO KNOW

1. colostomy
2. urinary incontinence
3. Diarrhea
4. flatus
5. catheter
6. micturition, voiding, urination
7. Catheterization
8. fecal impaction
9. enema
10. Constipation
11. defecation
12. fecal incontinence
13. Flatulence
14. ileostomy

TRUE AND FALSE

1. F — need not be reported
2. F — emptied immediately after each use
3. T
4. F — kept below the level of the
5. T
6. F — is not the same
7. F — with or without catheters
8. F — Not all clients will have a bowel movement every day.
9. F — low in residue
10. F — is a permanent or temporary bladder
11. T

MULTIPLE CHOICE

1. 1000 to 1500 ml
2. more
3. less
4. 600 ml
5. a disinfectant
6. smaller
7. stand
8. infection
9. at regular intervals
10. black
11. tarry
12. onions
13. fecal impaction
14. whenever it becomes soiled
15. ileostomy

CHECKING UP ON PROCEDURES

Giving the Client the Bedpan: 5, 1, 4, 3, 2
Catheter Care: 2, 5, 1, 3, 4
Emptying a Urinary Drainage Bag: 2, 3, 1, 4, 6, 5
Caring for the Client with a Colostomy: 4, 2, 6, 1, 5, 3

EQUIPMENT LIST

The following items need to be circled:
1. cotton balls
2. alcohol packets
3. soap and basin of water 4. bedpan

RECORDING AND REPORTING

Items marked with an "X": 2, 5, 6, 8, 9, 10.* (*It may be normal for a client to urinate during the night, however, this should be reported to determine if a problem exists.)

HIDDEN WORD SEARCH

1. B(E)D P A N
2. A P P(L)I A N C E
3. D E F A C A T(I)O N
4. C O M(M)O D E
5. R E S(I)D U E
6. E(N)E M A
7. K A R(A)Y A
8. O S(T)O M Y
9. M I C T U R(I)T I O N
10. S U P P(O)S I T O R Y
11. U R I(N)A L

Hidden word: ELIMINATION

CHAPTER 16: Collecting Specimens

TERMS TO KNOW

1. c
2. e
3. f
4. a
5. d
6. b

TRUE AND FALSE

1. F — You may not use the same container
2. T
3. F — also called the random urine sample
4. F — may be collected at any time
5. T
6. F — before the client voids
7. F — the first voiding is discarded; the last one is kept
8. T
9. F — the stone only needs to be sent
10. T
11. F — may not contain
12. T

MULTIPLE CHOICE

1. cool
2. 30
3. pancreas
4. four times
5. Fresh-fractional
6. 5 drops
7. sugar and acetone
8. early in the morning
9. water
10. labeled with the client's personal information

CHECKING UP ON PROCEDURES

Collecting a Clean-catch Urine Specimen: 3, 6, 4, 1, 5, 2
Collecting a Urine Specimen from an Infant: 1, 4, 2, 5, 3
Testing Urine: Testape: 2, 6, 4, 1, 3, 5
Testing Urine: Clinitest: 4, 2, 5, 1, 3
Testing Urine: Keto-Diastix: 2, 1, 5, 3, 4
Collecting a Sputum Specimen: 5, 3, 6, 1, 4, 2

CROSSWORD PUZZLE

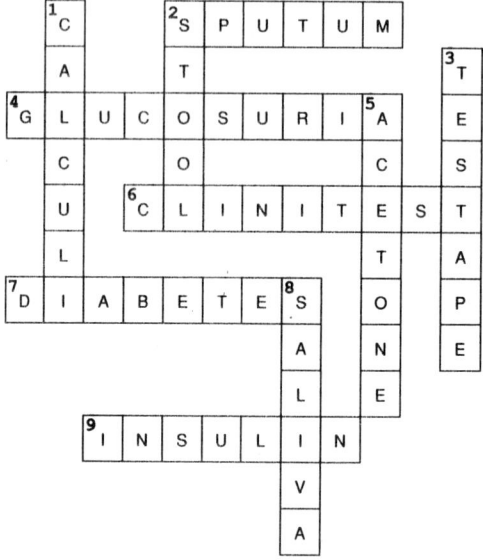

	1C		2S	P	U	T	U	M		
	A		T						3T	
4G	L	U	C	O	S	U	R	5I	A	
	C		O					C	S	
	U		6C	L	I	N	I	T	E	S	T
	L							T	A	
7D	I	A	B	E	T	8E	S	O	P	
						A		N	E	
						L		E		
			9I	N	S	U	L	I	N	
						V				
						A				

CHAPTER 17: Foods and Fluids

TERMS TO KNOW

1. nutrition
2. dehydration
3. intake
4. anorexia
5. dysphagia
6. output
7. calorie
8. edema
9. nutrient

TRUE AND FALSE

1. T
2. F — high in protein
3. F — include fruits, vegetables, breads, cereals, and sugar
4. F — and cannot be produced by the body
5. T
6. T
7. F — may have
8. T
9. F — Oxygen is (water is the second most important)
10. T
11. F — is allowed
12. F — milliliters or cubic centimeters

ANSWERS TO CHAPTER QUESTIONS

MULTIPLE CHOICE

1. protein
2. 9
3. strawberries
4. D
5. 2 to 3
6. decreases
7. 3000 mg
8. bland
9. carbohydrate
10. weekly
11. largest
12. 10
13. moist
14. spoon
15. 2
16. dehydration
17. midnight

FILL IN

Food Group	Examples of Foods	Servings (Adult)	Nutrients
Milk/dairy	Milk, cheese	2 cups	Proteins, fat, carbohydrates, calcium, riboflavin
Meat/fish	Beef, fish Poultry Peanut butter	2 or more	Proteins, fat, iron, thiamin
Fruit/veg.	Fruits, green and yellow vegatables	4 or more	Vitamin A, C;
Bread/cereal	Bread, cereal, pasta	4 or more	Proteins, carbohydrates B vitamins

CHECKING UP ON PROCEDURES

Feeding the Client: 4, 2, 1, 3, 5

MATCHING

Part 1.
1. d
2. e
3. b
4. a
5. c

Part 2.
1. c
2. e
3. d
4. a
5. b

LIST

1. cubic centimeter
2. intravenous
3. nasogastric tube
4. total parenteral nutrition
5. intake and output
6. milliliter
7. nil per os (nothing by mouth)
8. force fluids

HIDDEN WORD SEARCH

1. EXCHA(N)GES
2. MEN(U)
3. PRO(T)EIN
4. DEHYD(R)ATION
5. M(I)NERALS
6. FA(T)S
7. V(I)TAMINS
8. CARB(O)HYDRATES
9. I(N)TAKE

Hidden word: NUTRITION

CHAPTER 18: Special Procedures

TERMS TO KNOW

1. over-the-counter drug
2. constrict
3. medication
4. prescription drug
5. dilate
6. side effect

TRUE AND FALSE

1. T
2. F — may NOT be given
3. F — at body temperature
4. T
5. T
6. F — Home health aides may or may not be allowed to apply either hot or cold.
7. F — increases
8. T
9. F — Cold applications are
10. T

ANSWERS TO CHAPTER QUESTIONS

MULTIPLE CHOICE

1. route
2. topical
3. Sublingual
4. capsule
5. 4
6. nasal cannula
7. Heat
8. moist
9. 20
10. Sitz bath
11. higher
12. hot water bottle
13. dry
14. 5
15. 25

CHECKING UP ON PROCEDURES

Assisting with Medications: 4, 1, 2, 5, 3
Applying an Ice Bag: 2, 4, 3, 1, 5

EQUIPMENT LIST

The following items need to be circled:
1. large basin with cold water
2. large basin with ice
3. bath thermometer

LIST

1. a. Right client
   b. Right medication
   c. Right time
   d. Right route
   e. Right dose

2. a. Body temperature is normal or slightly over normal
   b. Shivering
   c. Cyanosis (bluish color of the skin)
   d. Other signs and symptoms of cold

3. a. every day
   b. every 6 hours
   c. four times a day
   d. after meals
   e. two times a day
   f. when necessary
   g. every other day

4. a. pain
   b. excessive redness
   c. blisters

5. a. pain
   b. burning
   c. blisters
   d. cyanosis (or pale, white, gray skin)
   e. shivering

CHAPTER 19: The Postoperative Client

TERMS TO KNOW

1. d
2. g
3. f
4. j
5. i
6. b
7. e
8. h
9. a
10. c

TRUE AND FALSE

1. T
2. F — refer any questions . . . to your supervisor
3. T
4. F — Not all clients will
5. T
6. T
7. F — is not responsible
8. T
9. F — may be painful
10. T
11. F — the lower part of the limb to the top
12. F — should be exposed

MULTIPLE CHOICE

1. incision
2. sterile
3. semi-Fowler's
4. open
5. 5
6. supine
7. abdominal support
8. scultetus
9. away from
10. twice
11. remove the stockings
12. two-thirds

CHECKING UP ON PROCEDURES

Coughing and Deep Breathing Exercises: 3, 4, 1, 5, 2
Applying Elastic Stockings: 5, 2, 1, 3, 4
Applying Elastic Bandages: 1, 4, 5, 3, 2

LABELING

FIG. 19–1. T binders

FIG. 19–2. Scultetus binder

FIG. 19–3. Breast binder

FIG. 19–4. Straight abdominal binder

CHAPTER 20: The Mother and Her Newborn

TERMS TO KNOW

1. sterilization
2. bubbling
3. rooting reflex
4. circumcision
5. umbilical cord

TRUE AND FALSE

1. T
2. T
3. F — Mothers may need to wash . . . with plain water.
4. F — from both breasts
5. F — Water
6. T
7. F — may need to burp
8. T
9. F — tub bath
10. T
11. F — cleaned with soap and water, or with baby wipes
12. T

MULTIPLE CHOICE

1. 3 months
2. 2 to 3 hours
3. calcium
4. 24 hours
5. 5 minutes
6. discarded
7. back
8. below
9. away from
10. 7 to 10 days
11. 100
12. football hold

CHECKING UP ON PROCEDURES

Sterilizing Bottles: 4, 2, 1, 3, 5
Diapering a Baby: 1, 4, 3, 6, 2, 5

LABELING

FIG. 20–1. Football hold
FIG. 20–2. Shoulder hold
FIG. 20–3. Cradle hold

LIST

1. crying or screaming for a long time
2. flushed, pale or perspiring
3. noisy, rapid, difficult, or slow respirations
4. coughing or sneezing
5. reddened or irritated eyes
6. turns the head to one side or puts a hand to one ear
7. skipped feedings
8. vomits most of the feeding or between feedings
9. passes hard, formed stools or watery stools
10. rash

CHAPTER 21: Common Health Problems

TERMS TO KNOW

1. Gangrene
2. tumor
3. benign tumor
4. malignant tumor
5. fracture
6. Amputation
7. closed fracture
8. compound fracture
9. Metastasis
10. stroke

TRUE AND FALSE

1. T
2. T
3. F — Open reduction . . . involves surgery
4. F — A wet cast is slightly forward for
5. F — Intermittent
6. T
7. F — abducted
8. F — encouraged to avoid bedrest
9. T
10. T
11. T
12. F — prefers to sit upright and
13. T
14. T
15. F — has too much insulin

MULTIPLE CHOICE

1. skin care
2. mouth
3. Osteoarthritis
4. 24 to 48 hours
5. should not
6. palms of your hands
7. skeletal
8. top to bottom
9. unoperated
10. calcium
11. higher
12. amplified
13. be washed daily
14. white
15. a heart attack
16. insulin shock

MATCHING

1. i
2. e
3. g
4. h
5. a
6. b
7. d
8. j
9. c
10. f

ANSWERS TO CHAPTER QUESTIONS

LIST

1. a. a change in bowel or bladder habits
   b. a sore that does not heal
   c. unusual bleeding or discharge from a body opening
   d. a lump or thickening in the breast or other body part
   e. difficulty swallowing or indigestion
   f. an obvious change in a wart or mole
   g. nagging cough or hoarseness
2. Any five of the following: pain, swelling and a tight cast, pale skin, cyanosis, odor, inability to move the fingers or toes, numbness, temperature changes, drainage on or under the cast, chills, fever, nausea and vomiting.
3. a. Face the client, call by name each contact, use familiar name, state your own name and show name tag.
   b. Tell client time and date each day; keep calendars and clocks with large numbers around the house; maintain day/night cycle; remind of holidays, birthdays, and special days; discuss current events.
   c. Follow familiar routine, do not rearrange furniture or belongings, be consistent, stay calm, relaxed, promote a peaceful atmosphere.
   d. Give short, simple, clear answers and instructions, explain before performing any task, allow time for client to answer.
4. a. unexplained weight loss   c. increased thirst
   b. increased urine production   d. hunger

CROSSWORD PUZZLE

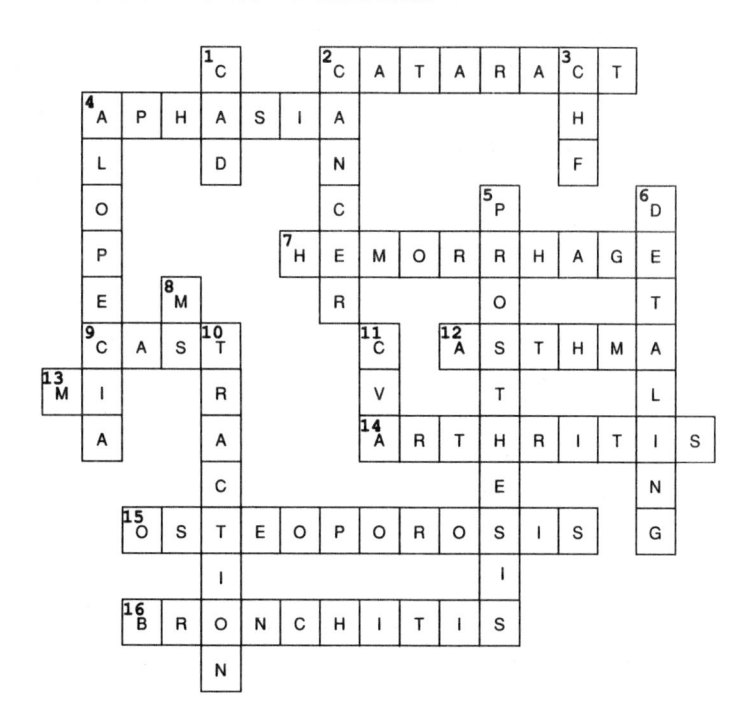

Across:
2. CATARACT
4. APHASIA
7. HEMORRHAGE
9. CAST
12. ASTHMA
14. ARTHRITIS
15. OSTEOPOROSIS
16. BRONCHITIS

Down:
1. COPE
2. CANCER
3. CHF
4. ALOPECIA
5. PROSTATE
6. DIABETES
7. HERNIA
8. M
10. TRACHA
11. CVA
12. A
13. MIA
15. OI

CHAPTER 22: Basic Emergency Care

TERMS TO KNOW

1. d
2. i
3. f
4. h
5. c
6. a
7. e
8. j
9. g
10. b

TRUE AND FALSE

1. F — do not move the victim
2. T
3. F — Respiratory arrest can occur without cardiac arrest.
4. T
5. F — carotid pulse
6. F — it is effective
7. T
8. F — a vein
9. T
10. F — immersed in cool water

MULTIPLE CHOICE

1. warm
2. cardiac arrest
3. is not
4. supine
5. lower
6. straight
7. 1 1/2 to 2
8. 80 to 100
9. 2
10. 5
11. two to three fingers
12. clutch at the throat
13. upward
14. direct pressure over
15. Grand mal
16. 10 to 20 seconds
17. should not
18. wet dressing or sheet
19. 5
20. affected

CHECKING UP ON PROCEDURES

Adult CPR: One Person: 5, 3, 2, 4, 1, 6
Clearing the Obstructed Airway: Unconscious Adult: 3, 1, 2, 5, 6, 4
Obstructed Airway: Finger Sweep Maneuver: 3, 1, 4, 5, 2

ANSWERS TO CHAPTER QUESTIONS

LIST

1. a. your location including street, city, and phone; add names of cross streets or roads, landmarks if possible
   b. tell what happened
   c. how many people need help
   d. give the condition of the victim(s), obvious injuries, life-threatening situations
   e. what aid is being given
2. a. Airway
   b. Breathing
   c. Circulate
3. a. LOOK at the victim's chest for rises and falls.
   b. LISTEN for escape of air.
   c. FEEL for the flow of air.
4. a. low or falling blood pressure
   b. rapid, weak pulse
   c. cold, moist, pale skin
   d. rapid respirations
   e. thirst
   f. restlessness
   g. confusion and eventual loss of consciousness

HIDDEN WORD SEARCH

1. H(E)IMLICH
2. VO(M)ITUS
3. HEMIPL(E)GIA
4. PA(R)AMEDICS
5. LO(G)ROLL
6. (E)MS
7. CHOKI(N)G
8. SUI(C)IDE
9. C(Y)ANOTIC

Hidden word: EMERGENCY

CHAPTER 23: The Dying Client

TERMS TO KNOW
1. reincarnation
2. terminal illness
3. autopsy
4. postmortem
5. living will
6. coroner
7. rigor mortis

TRUE AND FALSE
1. T
2. F — legal documents in some states
3. F — If your client does not have a DNR order,
4. T
5. F — Not all dying clients go through all five stages.
6. F — Hearing is
7. T
8. T
9. T
10. T

MULTIPLE CHOICE
1. 3
2. anger
3. Bargaining
4. denial
5. more
6. rises
7. semi-Fowler's
8. falls
9. your supervisor
10. before
11. 2 to 4 hours
12. never

CHECKING UP ON PROCEDURES
Postmortem Care: 6, 2, 4, 1, 5, 3

LIST
1. a. denial
   b. anger
   c. bargaining
   d. depression
   e. acceptance
2. a. Movement, muscle tone, and sensation are lost.
   b. Peristalsis and other gastrointestinal functions slow.
   c. Circulation fails and body temperature rises.
   d. Respiratory system fails, "death rattle" may be heard.
   e. Pain decreases, client loses consciousness.
3. a. no pulse
   b. no respiration
   c. no blood pressure
   d. pupils are fixed and dilated

Answers to Final Examination Questions

1. d	26. c	51. d	76. c
2. a	27. b	52. b	77. b
3. b	28. d	53. b	78. b
4. c	29. c	54. d	79. a
5. c	30. a	55. b	80. c
6. b	31. c	56. b	81. c
7. d	32. a	57. c	82. d
8. a	33. a	58. d	83. a
9. c	34. c	59. b	84. d
10. d	35. b	60. d	85. d
11. a	36. a	61. d	86. c
12. d	37. c	62. d	87. b
13. a	38. c	63. c	88. c
14. c	39. a	64. c	89. d
15. d	40. b	65. a	90. c
16. a	41. d	66. d	91. b
17. b	42. b	67. a	92. d
18. a	43. d	68. d	93. c
19. c	44. a	69. d	94. a
20. d	45. b	70. b	95. b
21. b	46. d	71. c	96. d
22. a	47. a	72. a	97. a
23. b	48. b	73. d	98. c
24. d	49. b	74. a	99. a
25. a	50. b	75. a	100. b

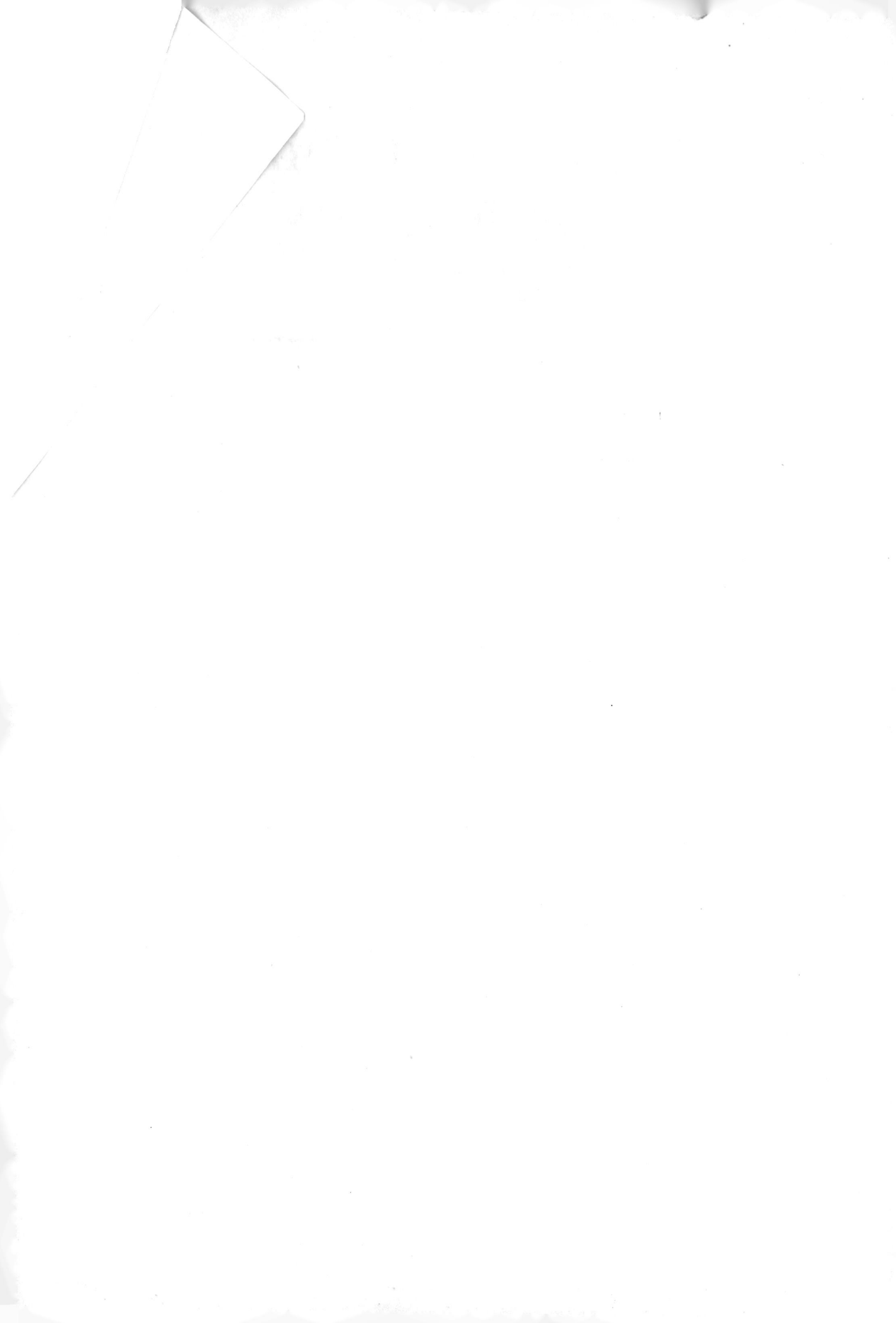